Neurology in Primary Care

Neurology in Primary Care

Joseph H. Friedman, M.D.

*Professor, Department of Clinical Neurosciences, Brown
University School of Medicine, Providence, Rhode Island;
Adjunct Professor, School of Pharmacy, University of
Rhode Island, Providence; Chief of Neurology, Memorial
Hospital of Rhode Island, Pawtucket*

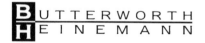

Boston   Oxford   Johannesburg   Melbourne   New Delhi   Singapore

Every effort has been made to ensure that the drug dosage schedules within this text are
accurate and conform to standards accepted at time of publication. However, as treatment
recommendations vary in the light of continuing research and clinical experience, the
reader is advised to verify drug dosage schedules herein with information found on prod-
uct information sheets. This is especially true in cases of new or infrequently used drugs.

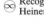 Recognizing the importance of preserving what has been written, Butterworth–
Heinemann prints its books on acid-free paper whenever possible.

 Butterworth–Heinemann supports the efforts of American Forests and
the Global Re-Leaf program in its campaign for the betterment of trees,
forests, and our environment.

Library of Congress Cataloging-in-Publication Data
Friedman, Joseph H.
    Neurology in primary care/ Joseph H. Friedman
        p.   cm.
    Includes bibliographical references and index.
    ISBN 0-7506-7036-3
    1. Nervous system--Diseases. 2. Neurology. 3. Primary care
(Medicine) I. Title.
    [DNLM: 1. Nervous System Diseases--diagnosis. 2. Primary Health
Care. WL 141F911n 1999]
RC346.F75 1999
616.8--dc21
DNLM/DLC
for Library of Congress   98-39867
                                                                    CIP

British Library Cataloguing-in-Publication Data
A catalogue record for this book is available from the British Library.

The publisher offers special discounts on bulk orders of this book.
For information, please contact:

Manager of Special Sales   For information on all B-H
Butterworth–Heinemann   publications available, contact our
225 Wildwood Avenue   World Wide Web home page at:
Woburn, MA 01801-2041   http://www.bh.com
Tel: 781-904-2500
Fax: 781-904-2620

10 9 8 7 6 5 4 3 2 1

Printed in the United States of America

In memory of my father,
who would have preferred a more scholarly book
with lots of references

Contents

Preface

This book provides a practical overview of the neurologic problems common in adult primary care medicine. It is meant to be useful and readable. It is not a textbook or encyclopedia of neurology. The standard textbooks of medicine generally have detailed and thoughtful discussions of the major neurologic disorders, which tend to be disease oriented and emphasize pathophysiology and treatment. This monograph, while including some discussions of particular diseases, primarily focuses on syndromes. I hope it provides a framework for approaching any patient with a neurologic problem. It should help the primary care provider conceptualize the problem, determine a reasonable course for evaluation and treatment, and know when expert help is required.

The most common neurologic problems for both the primary care provider and the neurologist are headache, dizziness, and back pain. In most cases the neurologist does little more than confirm the diagnosis of a migraine or tension headache, backache without nerve entrapment, or dizziness of unclear etiology, without "curing" the symptom. This may be a perfectly adequate use of the neurologist's expertise, reassuring the primary care provider and the patient that nothing more serious is wrong. However, in the era of managed care and shrinking resources, a referral to a neurologist is becoming more of a luxury than a right. In areas where neurologists are in short supply, appropriate restriction of referrals will enhance the usefulness of these specialists and help the primary care provider feel a greater sense of control. As the number of physicians in the United States trained as specialists declines, and managed care restricts patient access to them, an even greater reliance on the primary care provider will be required.

Although I am a subspecialist neurologist with a particular clinical and research interest in Parkinson's disease and movement disorders, I have also practiced general neurology since I completed my training in 1982. I have run the consult service of an adult general hospital since that time and have also been the neurologist for the Brown University Student Health Service since the spring of 1983. It was in that role that I had the idea for this book. After noticing that 75% of referrals were for the evaluation of headache, I gave what I consider to be the most effective lecture of my career. I spoke to the student health doctors, nurses, and physician's assistants on the diagnosis and management of headaches. The content of that talk is contained in the headache chapter in this volume. It diminished my referrals by 50%, reducing the wait for students to see me and simultaneously improving the quality of care I provided.

This book is not intended to reduce the role of the neurologist but rather to make the primary care provider better prepared and more confident in a field that many physicians approach with trepidation.

There is an old joke about two men walking down a path when a large frog hops in front of them and says, "Kiss me and I'll turn into a neurologist." One man bends down and the puts the frog in his pocket. The other turns to him and says, "Aren't you going to kiss him?" "No," he replies, "a talking frog is worth more than a neurologist." Well, if you ask the right questions, a neurologist may be worth a lot more than a talking frog. You can save on excessive testing and aggravating delays in diagnosis and treatment. I hope this small book will help.

JOSEPH H. FRIEDMAN

Acknowledgments

For their helpful criticism, I thank Peter Hollmann, M.D.; Brian Ott, M.D.; Sydney Louis, M.D.; George Paulson, M.D.; Bernard Zimmerman, M.D.; George Sachs, M.D.; John Nutt, M.D.; Mark Jacobs, M.D.; and John C.M. Brust, M.D. I also thank Mary Eddy for her expertise and perseverance in manuscript preparation.

1

Headache

There are two major classifications for headaches: primary headaches and secondary headaches. Primary headaches are migraine, tension, combination migraine-tension, and cluster headaches. Secondary headaches have identifiable etiologies such as sinusitis, subarachnoid hemorrhage, and neoplasm. An alternative classification that is perhaps more useful is *serious* and *not serious* headaches. *Serious* headaches have potentially serious medical implications and must be diagnosed and attended to promptly. Serious headaches are quite rare. Headaches that are *not serious* occur in the vast majority of headache patients seen by the primary care provider as well as by the neurologist. Not serious does not mean that the headaches are of minor significance. They may be ruining someone's life (although usually the severity of the headache is a reflection of other problems in the patient's life), but they will not cause harm outside of the pain itself.

Serious headaches have an organic etiology (Table 1.1) such as a tumor, infection, ruptured aneurysm, brain abscess, obstructive hydrocephalus, sinusitis, or temporal arteritis. Probably 99% of headaches seen by the primary care provider, however, are tension, migraine, or some combination of the two.

Headache may be the single most common reason for referral to a neurologist because it is an extremely frequent complaint. Headaches are also a common reason for emergency room treatment. About 5% of Americans suffer from daily headaches, and more than 70% suffer headache at some time. Usually a neurologist examines the patient who has a long history of headaches. If brain imaging has been unrevealing, electroencephalography and a panoply of blood studies have been normal, and trials of multiple

1

Table 1.1.   Warning signals for serious headaches

New-onset headaches in an adult
Slowly progressive headaches in an adult
Focal neurologic signs or symptoms (e.g., hemiparesis, field cut, aphasia)
Weight loss, fatigue, fever, stiff neck, rash, or other evidence of systemic
    illness
Headache in patient with cancer, acquired immunodeficiency syndrome,
    or immunosuppression
Sudden onset
Papilledema
Unilateral headache, always on the same side

medications have been unhelpful, neurologists are helpful only in confirming to the patient that the illness, while troubling, is not life-threatening. Sometimes a neurologist, perhaps to fortify the aura of the specialist, goes on to perform a variety of unneeded tests, such as magnetic resonance imaging (MRI) or electromyogram (EMG), to further convince the patient of the benign nature of the illness.

Headache refers to pain within the cranial vault, where the brain lies, and is distinguished from face pain. Headache pain is an interesting phenomenon because the brain itself is pain free. For example, brain surgery is sometimes performed under local anesthesia while the subject is fully awake. Structures giving rise to headache pain include the bones of the head and all its covers, parts of the dura, the first three cervical nerves, and the arteries within the dura and arachnoid. Most patients with headaches cannot localize their pain sufficiently to identify a focal source. Even when localized, most headache pain cannot be placed in a physiologic distribution.

Headaches are most common in younger adults and tend to decrease in severity and frequency after middle age. Migraines and tension headaches affect women more than men.

The most important aspects of a patient's history of headaches are the duration of the illness (i.e., age at onset); the distribution and quality of the pain; the frequency of the individual attacks; the length of the individual attack; the associated or warning phenomena (aura), such as nausea, vomiting, photophobia, scintillations, scotomata, and hemiparesis; and possible triggers, including psychosocial factors.

It is typically the history rather than the examination that distinguishes malignant from benign headaches. Benign headaches, even if increasing in severity or frequency, tend to be chronic and often started decades ago. New headaches in an adult are always a cause for concern. What few patients understand is that, with the exception of a ruptured aneurysm and meningitis, headaches from malignant processes, such as neoplasms, tend to be less severe than the usual pain reported by migraineurs or patients with tension headaches. A neurologist identifies a worrisome headache as a newly developed, slowly worsening headache that seems to be generally present and hinders function but does not prevent it.

Headaches of a new type that are present for weeks must always induce a search for a cause. Positional headaches that occur only with certain postures or are reliably relieved in certain positions that suggest blockage of an outflow track either in the brain's ventricles or in the sinuses should raise concern and trigger a request for a computed tomography (CT) scan of the brain or sinuses. The common syndromes of tension headache and migraine, however, require far more tact, judgment, and clinical art to treat. The malignant headache requires diagnosis, which is usually not a difficult problem once the potential gravity is understood. Treatment is also usually straightforward.

The patient's history must assess all the potential explanations for the headache. Most important for assessing the subacute headache are systemic symptoms and signs such as fever and weight loss. Sinus problems such as purulent nasal discharge, foul breath, previous sinus infections, pain with pressure changes, and facial pain should be explored. Dental problems such as broken dentures or teeth may indicate bruxism or excess teeth grinding. Pain after chewing suggests a temporomandibular joint problem. I ask general questions about changes in work, athletic, social, and academic performance associated with the headache, as these are more sensitive measures of overall function than the routine neurologic evaluation. Whereas changes in activities of daily living do not distinguish cause and effect, they are markers for severity. For example, I would not expect a brain tumor to cause headache without affecting functioning of everyday life because tumors generally do not cause headache until they are large. By the time headaches occur, either focal symptoms are present or subtle losses of function with increased lassitude and weight loss occur. Even depression, frequently associated with tension headaches, is not very severe if everyday function is spared. Certain populations, such as patients with human immune deficiency virus (HIV), those with a history of cancer, the demented, and the elderly, require special concerns. The elderly are at risk for subdural hematomas, HIV-positive patients are at risk for infections, and the demented are simply challenging to interpret.

TENSION HEADACHES

The evaluation for a presumed tension headache depends on the circumstance. A decades-long headache requires no testing. A decades-long headache that has recently become much worse over a few weeks may require a brain CT scan if no evidence of increased stress is unearthed. New (a few weeks old) tension headaches require a brain CT scan to settle the issue and exclude tumor. MRI scans are not necessary because any lesion big enough to cause a headache can be seen on a CT scan. An electroencephalogram (EEG) is never indicated for assessing headache.

In many patients it is impossible to distinguish between the chronic tension and migraine headache, or to label the three or four different headache syndromes the patient has. There is a wide variety of tension headache syndromes, but the most common is a squeezing pain over the entire scalp, often affecting the bifrontal region the most. It may be described as a feeling of pressure or weight or a sensation as if the head is expanding and is going to explode. There is no aura, and the pain simply begins as a minor discomfort. It often originates in the back of the neck (hence the concept of muscle tension as the etiology), then radiates up over the posterior scalp and either around the temples or over the top of the head before encompassing the entire head. Frequently, patients trace the distribution of the pain from one spot where it begins along a path that meanders considerably. Sometimes there is a lateralizing predominance to the pain's location, but it generally involves both sides. Bilateral head pain usually suggests a diffuse, nonfocal process. The pain is often present all of the time but has variable intensity. It does not awaken the patient but is present on awakening. Pain medications reduce the severity for a while until resistance develops, and ultimately nothing short of narcotics is helpful. Pain often worsens during the day but rarely precludes working or chores. Nausea, vomiting, visual changes, and focal neurologic deficits are absent. No systemic disease is present and the patient frequently has a depressed affect. A patient might say, "What do you expect? I've had this headache for 10 years!"

James Lance, a noted Australian neurologist and headache expert, comments that it "is deceptively easy to think of all patients with tension headaches as having an inadequate personality." But Lance proceeds to caution against overgeneralization. He notes that about one-third of tension headache sufferers are depressed. To put numbers on these generalizations, I include the following data from Lance's series: Eighty to ninety percent have bilateral head pain. Forty percent have a family history of some type of headache, and 18% have a family history of migraine. About 15% report that headaches began before the age of 10. Alcohol sometimes improves these headaches, which is not the case for vascular headaches. These patients' responses to non-narcotic pain relievers frequently result in chronic use of and difficulty withdrawing from the pain relievers. In Lance's series, more than 75% of 466 patients attending a headache clinic had headaches every day.

Tension headaches are often present in patients who also suffer migraines. Many patients will distinguish their usual headaches from their migraines, but in fact, in a fair percentage of cases, little separates the two except the severity of the pain. Some will have throbbing pain with nausea or visual aura that clearly distinguishes the syndromes. Tension headaches may be associated with mild photophobia or nausea, but these symptoms seem to be almost omnipresent, not episodic. The patient with tension headache and chronic photophobia wears sunglasses indoors and out and often appears depressed. The chronically nauseated tension headache patient tends to be gaining, rather than losing, weight, hampered from doing anything either social or physical by the headache. Lance suggests that the patient also be questioned about jaw pain, teeth clenching, denture breaking, and other stigmata of excessive muscle tension to more clearly exclude this as a cause.

The etiology of tension headache pain is unknown. For many years, a muscle contraction component helped form a popular hypothesis. This explained perhaps why muscle relaxants such as benzodiazepines or relaxation exercises were helpful. Unfortunately, studies of neck muscles have proved this theory untenable. Patients with tension headaches do not have excess posterior or scalp muscle contractions. (The examination, however, may reveal signs of excess muscular contraction. When asked to relax, patients frequently cannot. Their tone, assessed either by passive movements of the arms or neck, is increased, possibly even simulating a parkinsonian condition. The jaw cannot be let slack to allow the examiner to move it quickly up and down.) Although there are numerous studies of the psychic components of a tension headache briefly mentioned above, only a minority of patients can identify emotional precipitants. Some will note that the headaches began when they started a new job, their grown child moved back into the house, or some similar stressful event occurred, but this is not common.

Treatment

Breaking a decades-long headache syndrome is an enormous challenge. Even syndromes of shorter duration, perhaps only months long, are also difficult, often for different reasons. The relatively recent sufferer is far less likely to accept a diagnosis of tension headache. By the time such a patient sees a neurologist, frequently because the patient insisted on the referral to a subspecialist, there is an expectation that the consultation will lead to a diagnosis of an arcane syndrome, that something *was* wrong that the lesser authorities could not find. I usually try to defuse the delivery of my opinion by pointing out that there's no brain tumor or other seriously threatening problem. It is important to emphasize to the patient that the detailed examination and history taking reflected the seriousness with which the symptoms were evaluated. When I discuss tension headaches, I point out the importance of psychological state on pain perception. I note that there is the common expression "Joe's a pain in the neck" that indicates that even common usage refers to somatization of emotional stimuli. I also note that a soldier who might tolerate the loss of a limb in battle might, in a controlled setting, be unable to tolerate even minor pain like a splinter or a small cut.

Medications that have shown efficacy are amitriptyline and valproic acid. Depending on the patient's age, size, and estimated sensitivity to side effects, I recommend starting amitriptyline at 10–25 mg qhs and increasing weekly by the same amount at night to a maximum of 100 mg. When amitriptyline is not tolerated I try an alternative tricyclic, usually nortriptyline, with the same dose recommendations. The selective serotonin reuptake inhibitor paroxetine has also been advocated for various pain syndromes, but there are few data to support its use. Valproate, in the usual antiepileptic doses, may also be helpful and can be started as Depakote (the long-acting form), 250 mg bid and then increased if tolerated but inadequate. Analgesics often work, especially nonsteroidal anti-inflammatory drugs (NSAIDs), but once used on a chronic basis, they may be difficult to stop. This, by itself, is not a bad thing; after all, amitriptyline or valproate would be used daily too. The problem of increasing need often arises, however, at which point lowering or stopping the NSAID is difficult. Benzodiazepines may be considered, but the potential for depression and long-term abuse problems must be strongly considered.

Relaxation techniques should be considered for all patients with tension headache. These are best taught to the patient by a knowledgeable psychologist and consist of a series of exercises that allow the patient to obtain better control over excessive muscle contractions. Psychiatric or psychological consultation should be discussed when appropriate, and in refractory cases, referral to a headache or chronic pain center should be encouraged. These centers teach the patients how to live with their pain rather than cure it. The pain is moved from its central place in the patient's life to a less important place and is identified as an annoyance that must be dealt with, rather than allowed to control the victim's life.

MIGRAINE

The term *migraine* is frequently misused to identify a severe headache. The alternative synonym of *sick headache* for migraine is considerably more accurate. The definitions of the two migraine syndromes proposed by the International Headache Society are as follows. A *common migraine* is a recurrent headache, usually unilateral and associated with nausea, vomiting, photophobia, and sonophobia. *Classic migraine* or *migraine with aura* features episodic headaches preceded by a neurologic deficit, usually a visual disturbance involving both eyes, typically a scotoma or blurred area with spots or flashing lights, but possibly hemiparesis. Less common migraines are ophthalmoplegic migraine, involving weakness of one of the nerves supplying eye movements; retinal migraine, in which blindness occurs in a single eye; and acephalic migraine, a childhood syndrome of aura without headache.

The definition of migraine makes no mention of severity. Whereas there is a certain cachet to calling one's headache a migraine, there is none in having a tension headache. Many patients have no trouble in carrying the diagnosis of migraine but refuse the diagnosis of chronic tension headache. Patients, however, don't complain of mild headaches. They only seek medical attention if the headaches are severe or if the aura is worrisome.

Migraines are common, although less so than tension headaches. Surveys of large British and American general populations reveal a migraine prevalence of 16% in women and 10% in men. All studies show a female predominance and large variations with populations studied. Japanese industrial workers have a prevalence of 3%, whereas narcotic addicts in an Australian methadone clinic had rates of 21% in men and 45% in women.

Migraines generally begin in childhood or early adulthood and rarely start after age 50. There is a family history of migraines in about half of migraineurs. Because women are more affected, the mother is more likely to have the migraine and an affected sibling is more likely to be a sister.

Migraine Aura

Many migraineurs can predict a migraine within 24 hours through changes in appetite, mood, alertness, drowsiness, yawning, or thirst. These are considered premonitory symptoms and not auras. The aura is part of the migraine, in a manner analogous to an aura being part of a complex partial seizure. As in complex seizures, there can be an aura without a headache just as there are auras without seizures. Most auras are visual and arise from the visual cortex. They may be areas of blurring or grayness, distorted images, or colored or white spots. Zig-zag lines, called *fortification spectra*, may appear, followed by areas of scotomata. Other neurologic symptoms such as paresthesia, aphasia, olfactory and gustatory hallucinations, or sensory distortions are rare but well described. Their occurrence should always raise the question of an alternative diagnosis, unless regularly associated with typical headaches, such as seizure phenomena, which are also often followed by headaches. Migraine auras last 20–45 minutes, considerably longer than the aura of a seizure, and are then followed by the headache. Some auras can last as long as an hour.

Migraine Headache

Although we think of migraine as a vascular phenomenon, the pain is often constant rather than throbbing, or varies from one to the other. For unknown reasons, the hemicranial head pain associated with focal symptoms is mostly ipsilateral, rather than contralateral, to the symptoms. Nausea associated with the headache occurs in 90% of patients, and 75% of patients will sometimes vomit with an attack. The headache duration is extremely variable but is usually measured in hours. Persistence of headache for 72 hours without a 4-hour interruption during waking hours is termed *status migrainous.* The pain may be intolerably severe and require visits to an emergency room for narcotics, or it may be mild and responsive to over-the-counter analgesics. Pain is often accentuated by any sensory stimuli, such as light and sound.

Migraine Precipitants

What induces migraines is extremely variable. In most cases the syndrome arises without apparent provocation. Sleep deprivation and hunger are well-known precipitants in some. Certain foods, particularly red wine, champagne, and chocolate, have been implicated. Very small double-blinded trials in subjects claiming chocolate or red wine sensitivity using carob in place of chocolate and colored vodka and flavoring in place of red wine have supported the connection. Extrapolating these data to induce all tyramine-containing foods has not been supported. Restricted diets have generally been unsuccessful in reducing migraines. Vasodilators like nitrates, barometric changes, head trauma, and stress may induce a migraine. Probably the most common precipitant is menstruation. Many women have monthly migraines associated with their periods.

Natural History

Migraines usually improve or even resolve by late middle age. Most female migraineurs stop having headaches on reaching menopause. Men generally stop having migraine headaches by middle age as well. Although occasional patients may first develop migraines at this age, the headaches tend to be less severe and less frequent.

Treatment

With the development of sumatriptan, migraine management has improved dramatically. In approaching treatment, the first question to be answered is whether the patient requires symptomatic or prophylactic treatment.

A clear drug of choice for treating symptomatic migraine is a triptan-family drug. It can be administered subcutaneously, nasally, or orally. The injected route is more effective and faster, but many patients have difficulty injecting themselves, and family members are also often unwilling or unable to give the shots. The injection of 6 mg helps more than 70% of recipients within 1 hour and is very well tolerated. Two-thirds of the responders have complete resolution of the pain. The 100-mg pill helps 50% of patients in 2 hours and 75% within 4 hours. A second injection of sumatriptan does not improve the yield after the first injection. Thus, a failure to improve after one shot of sumatriptan should not provoke a second attempt. The medicine is very well tolerated, except by patients with angina who are subject to infarction. Oral sumatriptan, in a 100-mg dose, may be repeated every 2 hours for two doses. Nasal spray is almost as effective as the injection.

The ergots are other migraine-specific drugs and have been used for several decades. Oral ergotamine is usually in pills that contain other medications as well, such as caffeine, acetaminophen, or aspirin. It works best when taken during the aura and before the actual pain begins. Once the headache starts, the oral form of ergotamine is less useful. Patients should be advised to carry tablets with them and to take two tablets at the onset of the aura and then one every 30 minutes until the syndrome resolves or a total of six tablets have been taken. As with sumatriptan, there are risks of infarction in patients with coronary ischemia. Dihydroergotamine is given either intravenously or as a nasal spray. When given orally, it may work better in conjunction with antiemetics such as metoclopramide and prochlorperazine.

One of the problems in treating patients with migraine is slowed peristalsis, which undoubtedly contributes to the nausea. When metoclopramide, which increases peristalsis, was given to migraine sufferers, increased absorption of medication led to the demonstration that aspirin can be effective in treating migraine, if absorbed. This might be considered a first line of treatment.

Other medications that can be considered when other drugs either fail or fail to be tolerated are intravenous lidocaine and chlorpromazine. If all else fails, narcotics will always treat the acute headache. However, this solution should only be used on a temporary basis for fear of inducing reliance or even addiction. In addition, many patients experience worsened nausea while on narcotics.

Prophylactic medication is used in patients whose headaches occur frequently enough to justify daily medication. The most commonly used medications have been beta adrenergic blockers—propranolol in particular—and tricyclic antidepressants. Methysergide has been used for this indication for several decades but not often due to its side effects. Calcium channel blockers such as verapamil have been used for the last decade, and valproic acid has also been approved for this indication.

Propranolol in doses as low as 60 mg daily is effective in reducing the frequency and severity of attacks. Nadolol (80–160 mg per day), atenolol (100 mg per day), timolol (10 mg twice per day), and metoprolol (200 mg per day) all have also been reported to improve migraine and may therefore be tried if propranolol is not tolerated. Amitriptyline (and probably other tricyclics) is particularly useful because it prophylaxes against both migraine and tension headache, and many people suffer both with equal severity. Amitriptyline needs to be initiated at a low dose, such as 10–25 mg daily, and increased by the starting amount each week to avoid side effects. Even at this low starting dose and slow titration, it is common for patients, even young adults, to stop after one or two doses and report, "It makes me feel like a zombie." Dry mouth, constipation, and orthostatic hypotension are other common adverse events with all the tricyclics. The "zombie" report, however, is relatively well confined to amitriptyline alone.

CLUSTER HEADACHE

Cluster headache is a rare syndrome and is overdiagnosed. It is the only primary headache syndrome that has a male predilection, with a sex ratio of about 9 to 1. The onset is usually in the second or third decade of life, and the attacks are unlike other headache syndromes. Typical attacks occur in clusters of one to three headaches per day for 4 to 8 weeks at a time. Individual headaches last 20 minutes to 2 hours, but are usually on the shorter end. The pain is described as excruciating, like a drill applied to the eye. The pain tends to occur on the same side throughout the cluster bout. Frequently associated with the pain in an affected eye are unilateral tearing, unilateral nasal discharge, miosis, or mild ptosis. In some patients the pain attacks at a particular time of the day or during a particular time of the year. The only identified precipitant for headache attacks is alcohol, but this applies only to some patients at particular times. There is no familial association with migraines or even with cluster headache.

Treatment for cluster headache is varied. Some patients respond rapidly to breathing 100% oxygen, so they keep an oxygen canister at home. Prednisone, starting at 50–75 mg daily for 3 days with a slow taper until the headache disappears, is also used. Antimigraine medications such as methysergide, ergots, and sumatriptan are also helpful, although the ergots need to be given in advance of the headache.

SERIOUS HEADACHES

Headaches of a serious concern generally have one of the five following attributes: (1) recent onset and slow progression, (2) fever, (3) constitutional symptoms such as cough or weight loss, (4) sudden onset, and (5) new and different than previous headache syndromes (Table 1-2).

Subarachnoid Hemorrhage (Aneurysmal Hemorrhage)

The headache of a subarachnoid hemorrhage is described by some patients as the "sudden onset of the worst headache of my life." Also called a *thunderclap headache* because of the suddenness and severity of the attack, this headache is caused by rupture of the aneurysm. The aneurysm itself is pain free, even when large. These headaches

Table 1.2.   Types of headache

Serious Headaches	*Not Serious Headaches*
Brain tumor	Tension
Subarachnoid hemorrhage	Migraine
Temporal arteritis	Cluster
Meningitis	Post–lumbar puncture
Encephalitis	Viral syndrome
Sinusitis	Exercise induced
Brain abscess	"Ice pick"
Subdural hematoma	Ice cream
Subdural empyema	Caffeine withdrawal
Obstructive hydrocephalus	—
Intoxication	—
Pseudotumor cerebri	—
Glaucoma	—

are usually, but not always, debilitating. The mention of the hallmark features of a subarachnoid hemorrhage in chart notes requires appropriate testing to rule out a subarachnoid hemorrhage, including lumbar puncture if the CT scan is negative. Sometimes the initial hemorrhage is minor, causing a sudden but tolerable headache that goes unnoticed until a larger hemorrhage occurs, drawing attention to the earlier sentinel or herald hemorrhage. These initial hemorrhages are often not brought to medical attention and even when evaluated can easily be missed due to the absence of distinguishing symptoms or signs on examination. After a subarachnoid hemorrhage, most patients develop a stiff neck and fever. Both are due to an inflammatory response mounted against the blood irritants. The diagnosis of a subarachnoid hemorrhage is usually made with a CT scan, which shows blood (white areas) in the subarachnoid space at the base of the brain or in the sulci. About 10–15% of subarachnoid hemorrhages are not visualized on CT, so a lumbar puncture may need to be performed.

Brain Tumors

Surprisingly, brain tumors are not usually discovered as a result of headaches. Brain tumors usually come to attention as the result of progressive deficit, such as a hemiparesis, aphasia or field cut, or seizure. The typical headache associated with a brain tumor is a dull, aching pain, rarely severe, that began insidiously and seems to be always present. It often responds to low-level analgesics such as aspirin or acetaminophen. The melodramatic complaint of an "excruciating headache that is ruining my life" is rarely heard from a patient with a brain tumor.

Headache occurs if there is secondary hydrocephalus or if pain-sensitive structures are stretched. Tumors can grow extremely large without causing any headache. Small tumors are unlikely to cause pain; hence, an unenhanced brain CT scan is an adequate test for evaluating headaches because it is not likely to miss a tumor large enough to cause headaches.

Temporal Arteritis

Temporal arteritis is almost entirely restricted to patients in their seventies and is rarely reported in patients younger than 50. Patients generally suffer from temporal scalp tenderness and have jaw or tongue claudication. Constitutional symptoms such as fever, weight loss, weakness, and malaise are common. Headache is a common feature and is variable in nature, with pulsatile aching or boring pain and with variable intensity and frequency. There may be palpable swelling of the temporal artery. Markedly elevated erythrocyte sedimentation rates are the rule, only rarely misleading by being low. Biopsies are required for diagnosis. Because the risk of untreated temporal arteritis is loss of sight that is virtually never recovered, the clinical rule is to have a low threshold for biopsy and treatment, which must be done on an urgent basis. Temporal arteritis is commonly associated with polymyalgia rheumatica, but the two disorders are not identical.

Sinus Headaches

Sinus headaches usually localize to the face and are usually associated with symptoms of sinus disease such as purulent discharge, foul breath, and malodorous taste, as well as abnormal mucus, fever, and malaise.

EXERCISE-INDUCED HEADACHE

The syndrome of benign exertional headache was recognized by Hippocrates, who wrote "one should recognize those who have headaches from gymnastic exercises, or running, or walking." Such headaches have a pulsatile quality suggesting increased blood flow as the etiology. Patients recognize the association between the headache and exercise and come to medical attention to rule out a lesion, presumably a vascular malformation or neoplasm. Exercise-induced headache is a benign syndrome that requires only reassurance in most cases. If the pain always localizes to a single location, then an MRI scan is in order. The fears over an aneurysm or arteriovenous malformation are understandable but not founded. I saw a small number of college athletes who developed exercise-induced headaches shortly after using a new weight-lifting apparatus. How this caused headaches never was clear to me, but the temporal association was definite.

Treatment is with indomethacin, aspirin, or probably any NSAID given an hour or two before the exercise. The patients, usually healthy young adults, often just want reassurance and to continue their exercise program.

POST–LUMBAR PUNCTURE HEADACHE

After a lumbar puncture, about 10% of patients experience a headache. It is a dull ache that appears when the patient is sitting upright or standing and resolves when the patient is lying flat. It usually resolves in 1 or 2 days. Treatment, if required, is a blood patch, usually administered by an anesthesiologist. A small volume of the patient's blood is drawn and then injected epidurally at the site of the lumbar puncture, which presumably seals the dural hole.

HEADACHES DURING PREGNANCY

Most migraine syndromes do not worsen during pregnancy. Because most headache patients are female and many are fertile, the issue of headache treatment and pregnancy is very relevant in primary care. The most important approach is education that includes discussing with patients, in advance, the use of medication and possible pregnancy. Obviously, as few drugs as possible or none should be used in women who are either pregnant or attempting to conceive. In cases in which conception occurred while the woman was on medication, the obstetrician must be notified. Relaxation therapy and regular exercise are the treatments of choice.

Although the situation is not mentioned in texts on headache, obstetricians consider headaches a very common complication of the first trimester of pregnancy but do not get concerned unless they are particularly severe or fail to resolve by the second trimester.

NEUROLOGIC EXAMINATION

The single most important sign in evaluating headaches is papilledema. Patients will usually report neurologic problems, but papilledema cannot be appreciated by the patient.

CLINICAL PEARLS

- The American Academy of Neurology has stated that an EEG is not a useful test for evaluating headaches.
- A brain CT scan is sufficient for almost all headache evaluations. With rare exceptions, the MRI will not be more sensitive.
- Years-long headaches do not require brain imaging for evaluation.
- Migraine headaches with nausea should be treated by a nonoral route (injection, nasal spray, suppository) or absorption will be problematic.

- A migraine headache may not be severe.
- Tension and migraine headaches usually hurt more than headaches from brain tumors.
- A complaint of "the sudden onset of the worst headache of my life" requires a lumbar puncture if a CT scan does not reveal sub-arachnoid blood.
- Sudden-onset headaches may occur with blockage of a sinus.

2

Dizziness

Dizziness is a common complaint but virtually useless as a medical term. People use the term *dizzy* to refer to a wide variety of symptoms that typically include vertigo, presyncope, imbalance, mental fogginess, and a variety of nonspecific terms. Most dizzy patients sent to neurologists have presyncopal symptoms. Few have vertigo or brain stem symptoms.

Presyncopal dizziness is a feeling of lightheadedness or a feeling of being distant from the environment. Patients may become diaphoretic, nauseated, sleepy, or even transiently vertiginous. There may be an associated palpitation, shortness of breath, or chest pressure that points to a cardiac source of hypotension, but this is rare. Lightheadedness usually occurs when the patient is standing. Either the spell occurs shortly after standing up or after the patient has been standing for a long time. Hyperventilation also produces lightheadedness and may be part of a panic attack.

Imbalance is a term patients will frequently use to elaborate on the term *dizzy*. It usually refers to a problem with gait instability that may include cerebellar or sensory ataxia or drug intoxication from a variety of drugs including anticonvulsants, narcotics, or benzodiazepines. Imbalance occurs when standing, walking, or, occasionally, sitting.

Nonspecific symptoms, such as mental cloudiness or fogginess, feeling "like a balloon," thinking "I'm not all there," and so on, are other common descriptions used to explain the symptom of dizziness. These are much more difficult to interpret. Whereas lighthead-

Table 2.1.   Dizziness

Type	Nature	Mechanism
Presyncopal	Lightheadedness	Low blood flow
Vertigo	Spinning or moving	Labyrinthine or brain stem dysfunction
Foggy	Poor concentration, mental dullness, fogginess	Hypoglycemia; medication effect; psychogenic
Imbalance	Gait instability, poor balance	Impaired balance due to cerebellar disease, peripheral neuropathy, hypothyroidism, bilateral vestibular dysfunction

edness implies a cardiovascular problem and imbalance points to a neurologic or a neuro-otologic problem, these forms of dizziness have an unclear etiology unless attributable to medication or drug side effects. These symptoms are often interpreted as psychological in origin but may be ultimately explained by some systemic medical problem such as hypothyroidism (Table 2.1).

Vertigo refers to a sensation of movement, either in the environment or in the individual. Most commonly this is a sensation of spinning but can be a movement like a boat on water. Patients may feel motion sickness or seasickness. Patients feel off-balance and, if the onset is sudden while the patient is standing, he or she will describe the floor as suddenly coming up at him or her rather than describing a typical fall. Acute vertigo is the sensation we all experienced as children when we spun ourselves around quickly several times, then suddenly stopped. We then perceived the environment as spinning, and to keep from falling, we planted our feet far apart and put our arms out to steady ourselves and to protect against injury in case of a fall. (As an "experiment," have your child or coworker spin around until dizzy and then stop. Observe the eyes for the nystagmus and note that it resolves as the vertigo resolves.)

The history generally provides the most important data for diagnosis. Both presyncopal and vertiginous dizziness occur on standing.

The presyncopal feeling is due to orthostatic hypotension, whereas the vertigo is due to a change in the head position. Thus, vertigo will be triggered with head rotations while the patient is seated, which is not the case for orthostatic symptoms. Vertiginous patients will often state that when an attack occurs, they must keep their head still. If the patient lies down, it must be in a single position only, face up or a particular ear down. Turning over or sitting up produces symptoms. None of these positional changes cause symptoms for nonvertiginous dizziness. The other forms of dizziness are not exacerbated by changes in position. The imbalance form of dizziness occurs only in an unsupported position, typically standing or walking (i.e., not seated). Moving the head will worsen the sensation if the patient is standing but will not induce symptoms when the patient is seated in a chair.

EXAMINATION

Once the type of dizziness is determined from the history, the examination will focus on the appropriate organ system: cardiovascular, labyrinth, brain, or peripheral nerve. For cardiovascular dizziness, 1–3 minutes of pulse rates should be checked along with a cardiac examination and, most important, orthostatic blood pressure should be checked over the course of 3 minutes. Because the degree of orthostasis may vary considerably depending on volume status, medication effects, ambient temperature, and other factors, the office evaluation may not confirm an association between the symptoms and the blood pressure drop. A fall of 15 points systolic, especially if no compensatory rise in heartbeat occurs, supports a diagnosis of orthostatic hypotension from an autonomic neuropathy or overly aggressive beta-adrenergic blockade from medications.

Dizziness brought on by hyperventilation occurs in younger patients and can be safely reproduced in the office. Hyperventilation is uncomfortable and must be maintained for more than 1 minute, preferably for 2, to check if dizzy symptoms have been reproduced.

Imbalance is checked by observing the patient walk, preferably for a distance of 20 feet or more. Walking in a small examination room is not sufficient. One should look for a wide base, loss of balance to one side or another, or staggering from side to side. It should be remembered that mild dysfunction will not produce severe ataxia. As with any disorder, imbalance varies from mild to severe. Tandem gait is a more demanding test of balance than normal walking. The Romberg test, having the patient standing with feet together and eyes closed, is a test of balance. With unilateral cerebellar or unilateral inner ear dysfunction, the patient will lean or sway toward the side of the lesion. With midline cerebellar or bilateral inner ear dysfunction, the patient will sway randomly. The Romberg test is not a cerebellar test; it is a balance test. It was originally developed to test for tabes dorsalis, a form of tertiary syphilis, in which the posterior columns of the spinal cord are damaged so that position sense is lost. With the eyes closed and position sense absent, the patient no longer perceives direction or changes in direction once he or she starts to sway, which all people do. Not sensing the positional change, he or she would just fall to the ground if not caught. Another method of bringing out a subtle deficit is to have the patient march in place with eyes closed. A unilateral deficit, cerebellar or vestibular, will produce rotation.

To test for labyrinthine dysfunction, the examination should focus on eye movements. True vertigo is always associated with nystagmus. When the patient is symptomatic, nystagmus is observable. Nystagmus is the sudden jerking movement of the eyes that represents a rapid correction of a slow drift in the opposite direction. Nystagmus is labeled by the direction of the fast phase. It is usually horizontal, when it is left-beating or right-beating, but it also may be vertical or torsional. It may be defined further by when it occurs. If it occurs when the patient is looking to one side, it is called gaze-evoked nystagmus. *Positional nystagmus* is the term for nystagmus induced by changes in head position and may be sustained or transient. It should be noted that nystagmus is not perceived by the patient. Although an observer sees the patient's eyes jerking, the patient does not necessarily see the environment moving or feel his or her eyes moving. Nystagmus arises from peripheral (inner ear) or central (brain stem) origin. Clinically these can be distinguished by the following features: fixation, latency, fatigability, and directionality. An inner ear or vestibular nerve nystagmus is suppressed with fixation, so the patient is more comfortable with his or her eyes open. This is the reason ice skaters pick out objects to focus on when spinning to avoid vertigo. Fixation does not help central vertigo. With positional changes, peripheral lesions produce vertigo and nystagmus after a latency of 3–10 seconds, whereas central lesions produce immediate symptoms and signs. Peripherally induced nystagmus does not change direction with a change in gaze, but central nystagmus does. Finally, and least useful clinically, is the difference in fatigability. Peripheral lesions fatigue so that repeated head position changes produce less vertigo each time. Centrally induced vertigo does not habituate. It is a rare patient, however, who will permit repeated bouts of positionally induced vertigo. Cerebellar disease causes horizontal nystagmus in the direction of the gaze, more severe on the affected side if unilateral. Vestibular dysfunction typically induces torsional (rotary) nystagmus classified as clockwise or counterclockwise depending on the direction. This does not reverse direction so that the nystagmus will be clockwise or counterclockwise when looking left and right but becomes more severe when the patient is looking to the affected side. Should the patient become vertiginous during the examination, the physician should look at the eyes to confirm the presence of nystagmus.

I generally ask the patient to try to bring on the vertigo by shaking his or her head. If this does not suffice, a Hallpike maneuver may be attempted. The patient is slowly placed in a supine position with the head hanging over the exam table and kept in this position for about 1 minute. He or she is then sat up. After a few minutes' rest, the procedure is repeated but this time with the head turned 90 degrees to have one ear down. The maneuver is repeated with the other ear down. If vertigo occurs, the eyes should be examined for nystagmus. When bilateral vestibular dysfunction is present, this maneuver will not induce vertigo or nystagmus. In this case caloric testing can be tried. Caloric testing can also be used in unilateral disease. Small amounts of cold or warm water are instilled into the ear canal while the patient is lying flat and his or her head is inclined 30 degrees. Initially 0.2 ml of ice water should be used, then 0.5 ml before larger volumes are tested. The normal response of an intact vestibular system is given by the mnemonic COWS (cold opposite, warm same), which gives the direction of nystagmus after cold- and warm-water infusions. This is an extremely potent stimulus so that only small volumes should be used for the first attempt. For unilateral disease, a difference of 20% in the duration of the response is considered significant. For bilateral disease, a lack of response or a small response to a large volume of ice water is diagnostic.

More sophisticated testing requires special equipment. An electronystagmogram or posturography can be used to objectively and accurately measure labyrinthine response and should be available in an ear, nose, and throat office or at a university center.

Causes of Vertigo

Table 2.2 provides a summary of the causes of vertigo.

Ischemia is a rare cause of vertigo in general but more commonly occurs in the elderly. Vertigo may occur as a result of ischemia to the labyrinthine artery, affecting the labyrinth and auditory vestibular nerve in isolation or, more commonly, to the brain stem. The characteristic features are the occurrence with deafness of associated brain stem symptoms (diplopia, hemiparesis, hemianesthesia, and limb or speech ataxia), and the onset of symptoms occurs upon standing secondary to orthostatic hypotension or without any provocation at all (i.e., without a change in head position). The characteristic patient has the usual risk factors for cerebrovascular disease—namely, previous transient ischemic attacks (TIAs) or strokes, hypertension, diabetes, cardiac disease, or cigarette smoking. The proper evaluation for this cannot produce a definitive diagnosis and is probably best handled by a neurologist. Testing should include a brain magnetic resonance imaging (MRI) scan and either magnetic resonance angiography (MRA) or intracranial Doppler studies. The MRI will determine if previous, often unsuspected, strokes have occurred or whether the presumed TIA may represent a tumor or arteriovenous malformation. The Doppler study or

Table 2.2.   Causes of vertigo*

Causes	Age	Characteristics
Infectious or postinfectious	Adults	Acute onset; persists for days; viral association; occurs in mini-epidemics
Ménière's disease	Elderly	Associated with hearing loss and tinnitus
Benign positional vertigo	Elderly	Brief episodes occurring with head position changes
Post-traumatic	Any	Onset after trauma; persistent
Endolymphatic fistula	Elderly	Worsens with pressure changes
Ischemia	Elderly	Acute onset possibly related to orthostasis, not head position; associated with other brain stem symptoms; isolated vertigo in the elderly

*Note that all forms of vertigo worsen with changes of head position.

MRA will provide information on the major arteries, which is sometimes useful. Impending occlusion or significant stenosis may heavily weight a decision for anticoagulation, whereas a normal study may point to antiplatelet therapy. Endarterectomies are not performed in the vertebrobasilar territory, and angioplasty and stenting are still in their infancy and not yet of proved value.

One study of acute vertigo in the elderly identified vertebrobasilar insufficiency with infarction of the lower portion of the cerebellum in six of 24 patients above the age of 50 seen in an emergency room. There were no reliable distinguishing features between the brain ischemic group and the labyrinthine group. All patients had nystagmus, and only two of the six with cerebellar infarcts had typical direction-changing nystagmus on looking to either side. All evaluated patients had persistent vertigo, and none had other neurologic signs or history of inner ear problems. It was thus a skewed population but nevertheless contained a surprising result for neurologists: Such a high percentage of isolated prolonged vertigo without other symptoms can be caused by cerebellar infarction. Prolonged vertigo may therefore warrant a brain MRI scan in elderly patients.

Treatment

True vertigo is treated with symptomatic medications, such as meclizine, promethazine, and atropine patch, until the episode resolves. Special rehabilitation exercises are sometimes helpful as well.

CLINICAL PEARLS

- Hyperventilation as part of a panic attack may cause dizziness.
- Fainting is almost never the result of a central nervous system disorder.
- Fainting is not due to carotid stenosis.
- Vertigo from inner ear dysfunction is directly proportional to the degree of nystagmus.
- If the patient is vertiginous and no nystagmus is present, suspect a cerebellar etiology.
- Vertigo due to labyrinthine dysfunction is associated with nausea and its concomitants, as well as gait ataxia, but no other nervous system impairments.
- Vertigo is the sensation a person develops when he or she spins around several times and then stops.

3

Backache, Neckache, and Radiculopathies

Low back pain (LBP) is one of the major causes of neurologic referral as well as disability in the United States and other Western countries. Almost all people have had episodes of LBP, and about 10% of neurologic referrals are for evaluation of LBP. It is of some interest that doctor referrals for LBP are highly culturally dependent. While LBP is common in the Western world, it is a relatively uncommon cause for medical attention in parts of the Third World. Only a small fraction of patients seen by neurologists suffer from lumbosacral nerve entrapment and these represent an even smaller minority for the primary care physician (PCP). It is clear that pinched nerves are not the usual explanation for LBP. Pinched nerves are still, however, fairly common overall, and failure to recognize them leads to more suffering and a less happy outcome.

Diagnosing causes for LBP is difficult. Recognition of how prevalent spine abnormalities are underscores this fact. More than 85% of adults have autopsy-confirmed disk degeneration by age 50 and almost all elderly people have arthritis on spine x-rays. Thus, telling an adult older than 50 that he or she has arthritis or disk degeneration is almost always true, although these symptoms are often unrelated to back pain.

The spine consists of articular joints like other joints. The anterior part of the spine consists of the body of the vertebra, which bears the bulk of the body's weight. Disks sit between the bodies of the vertebrae. Posterior to the body of the backbone is the spinal cord, surrounded by bone parts that form the articulations between the levels, allowing the spine to bend. There are ligaments that hold the bones together as well as muscles attaching vertebrae to each other and to other bones. To envision the enormous force required to maintain the upright posture, one can think of the spine as the mast of a sailboat. The body's weight, like the sail of the boat, is anterior, pulling the spine or mast forward. Because the support is fixed at its base, a huge torque is created dependent on height, abdominal girth, and the geometry of its distribution.

The spinal cord travels within the spinal canal but ends at about the L1 vertebral body. Sensory and motor nerves exit at each segmental level and then travel downward with the cord until exiting the intervertebral foramen in the anterolateral space below the vertebral body of the appropriate nerve and fusing. The sensory nerve cell body is not in the cord; it sits outside the spinal cord. The spinal cord itself is pain-free, but the joints, muscles, periosteum of the bone, ligaments, and outer layer of the disk (annulus fibrosis) all carry pain fibers. Pain fibers from the sacroiliac joint enter the cord via the L5 and S1 roots.

Adams and colleagues note four types of LBP: local, referred, radicular, and secondary (protective). Local pain arises at the location where the pain is felt. Bone fractures, focal infections, and tumors stretching the periosteum or affecting joints, muscles, ligaments, and fascia cause local pain. The pain may be constant or transient, and may be relieved or exacerbated by mechanical changes. Referred pain may mimic nerve root pain by following the course of a nerve, or may also radiate in nondermatomal patterns (e.g., to the hip or to viscera). In addition, visceral pain may occasionally be referred to the spine. Radicular pain is due to nerve root compression. It may be present all the time or only with certain maneuvers. When constantly present, it tends to have an aching quality. With exacerbations, however, it is a sharp, stabbing, or electrical-like pain that shoots from the midline back along the course of the nerve, sometimes as far as the distal end of the nerve (e.g., to the lateral aspect of the foot with S1, or the dorsum of the great toe with L5), but often only part of the distance. Because this is usually due to a mechanical problem—that is, something like a disk fragment or arthritic spur pressing on the nerve—it worsens with maneuvers that increase intrathoracic pressure such as coughing or sneezing. Twisting, bending, or extending the leg increases

Table 3.1. Causes of back pain

Musculoskeletal
Developmental deficits of cord and spine
Neoplasm of spine, cord, or roots
Metabolic bone disorders
Infections

the pressure on the nerve by directly putting pressure on it. Paresthesias (tingling or "pins and needles") in the nerve distribution, aching in an innervated muscle, and isolated muscle cramps are common. Secondary pain is due to muscle spasm in the lower back, usually due to local irritation or a mechanical problem, such as kyphoscoliosis. A leg or foot problem may cause altered gait and posture, leading to lower spine pain with spasm. (This then leads to a chicken and egg–type problem for the clinician. Did the muscle spasm cause the gait and posture abnormality or vice versa?)

The causes of back pain, acute or chronic, are legion. Most causes are, as with other pain syndromes, medically benign, although frequently socially and functionally disastrous. However, the PCP must know when the red danger flag should go up. General causes of LBP are listed in Table 3-1, and signs or symptoms that should alert the PCP to a potentially serious problem are listed in Table 3-2.

Table 3.2. Indications of serious pain problems

Weight loss
Constitutional symptoms (fever, cough)
History of cancer
Progressive pain despite rest
Radicular pain that does not remit with positional changes
Focal weakness or sensory loss
New bladder dysfunction
New leg weakness
New gait dysfunction
Sensation of a belt or girdle around the trunk
Thoracic pain

NEUROLOGIC SYNDROMES

Neurologic syndromes are associated with nerve or spinal cord problems, usually recognizable as such by the patient's history and confirmed by examination.

Herniated Disk

It is generally not appreciated that herniated, ruptured, or "slipped" disks have an age predilection. Unlike arthritic diseases, which increase with age, herniated nucleus pulposus (HNP) peaks in the fourth and fifth decades. It is rare under age 25 and over age 60. In the elderly this is because the gelatinous inner portion of the disk solidifies over time, making the extrusion of disk core material less likely. The most common disk to herniate is between the fifth lumbar vertebra and the first sacral vertebral body. The next most commonly affected disk is between L4 and L5. Disk herniations are increasingly less likely as the lumbar level numbers ascend and the vast majority of disk herniations are at L5-S1 and L4-L5, with all others quite infrequent. There are no sacral disks; hence, there are no sacral disk herniations.

Pain from an HNP is generally of a sharp, stabbing nature, radiating along the affected nerve, typically S1 or L5, which run together in the sciatic nerve. This pain is generally superimposed on a chronic, more aching pain. Exacerbations occur with mechanical changes in the spine. Usually the pain starts in the spine and radiates to the buttock or leg in a sciatic distribution, but sometimes the back component of the pain is quite small. Patients may alter their posture when standing. Relief usually occurs from lying flat, by virtue of reducing the enormous torque on the lower spine caused by the maintenance of the upright posture, whether sitting or standing. Spinal muscle spasm may produce a second, local pain syndrome and induce scoliosis. Reducing pressure on the nerve entrapment is accomplished by relaxing the lower spine and by flexing the knee and hip. Patients generally lie in bed with the knee and hip flexed.

Although most HNPs compress S1 or L5, producing sciatic pain, higher roots or, rarely, multiple roots may be compressed. L4 root compression causes pain radiating to the anteromedial calf, L3 to the anterior medial thigh or groin, and L2 to the lateral hip. Occasionally lumbar root pain will radiate to the testicle and be evaluated as a urogenital problem.

Spinal Stenosis

Some people are born with narrower than normal spinal canals. While not problematic by itself, this condition leaves the cord and roots more vulnerable to processes that further narrow the canal, such as herniated disks or arthritic changes. Spinal stenosis is a syndrome that behaves like a claudication phenomenon.

Patients with spinal stenosis gradually develop weakness and numbness in their legs when standing or walking that is relieved by sitting. They find it particularly difficult to walk downhill. Symptoms may begin on one side and then spread to the other leg. If the patient can reproduce the symptoms, then the physician can actually detect focal weakness and deep tendon reflex changes during a brief period. Surgical widening of the lumbar canal can markedly improve the situation.

Vertebral Fractures

Vertebral fractures occur with severe trauma in normal individuals but with minor or even no trauma in people with osteoporosis, typically elderly women not taking estrogen. The pain is localized and unremitting. It does not radiate and generally takes weeks to resolve. In osteoporotic women, the fractures lead to height loss and exaggerated curvature. When several bones collapse the patient takes on the appearance of a person who is squeezed from above. Vertebral fractures cause abdominal discomfort due to the increased pressure on abdominal organs.

Back Strain and Back Sprain

Back strain and *back sprain* are ill-defined terms that encompass a large collection of clinical syndromes that are linked by historical similarities and lack of objective signs for diagnosis. One can easily explain the acute back injury when a patient experiences LBP after an injury or after lifting a heavy object in a disadvantaged manner. Many patients, of course, develop LBP simply on bending or turning, unrelated to the performance of any untoward activity. The pain is local, in the paraspinal region, but may radiate. The symptom of pain radiating across both sides of the lower back is helpful in that this symptom is not likely due to root disease (which is typically unilateral and radiates down one leg) and therefore implies a musculoskeletal etiology. However, the pain may radiate in a nerve distribution, but usually not.

The radiating nature of LBP in many patients is a major clinical challenge. This phenomenon is the most common precipitant for the referral to a neurologist or surgeon. In an often-cited experiment many years ago, an irritant was injected into the apophyseal joints of symptomatic and asymptomatic people, producing local and radicular pain, despite the lack of nerve root involvement. The most severe symptoms occurred in the already symptomatic patients. Confirmation of this result can be seen with the frequent relief of sciatic and other radicular symptoms when lidocaine or steroids are injected into a problematic spinal joint. Interestingly, paresthesias are frequently described and the pain sometimes travels in a nerve distribution. The explanation for this remains unknown.

Paraspinal muscle spasm may cause spinal curvature. Any movement may produce excruciating back pain but, unlike pain from a pinched nerve, there is no neurologic deficit.

Chronic Low Back Pain

Chronic LBP without neurologic disease is a much more challenging problem than acute LBP. Frequently charged with psychodynamic issues, such as litigation, disability, depression, and personality disorders, patients with chronic LBP are best treated in a behaviorally oriented chronic pain center once a complete evaluation has been performed. One of the difficulties in diagnosis is the very high rate of "abnormal" spine imaging studies.

Osteoarthritis

Osteoarthritis (OA) is used to explain most back pain syndromes that are not of traumatic or disk origin. Arthritic spurs in the foramen pinch nerve roots, causing symptoms indistinguishable from disk herniation, so that OA contributes to LBP by causing nerve root entrapment, arthritic joint pain, or both. As noted above, pain in a facet may radiate, causing difficulty distinguishing nerve root pain from radicular non-nerve pain. The distinction is important because management is different.

EVALUATING THE PATIENT

History

The patient's history may be more important than the examination. Slowly progressive back pain in the lumbar region or any pain in the thoracic spine (see the section on thoracic pain) should be cause for concern, particularly for neoplasm. Fever associated with spinal pain at any level, especially if focal, raises the issue of an infectious process. Epidural abscess is a medical emergency requiring surgical drainage and appropriate antibiotics after a culture is obtained.

Most back pain is acute and occurs with bending or twisting, particularly with lifting a heavy weight. Certain features in the history point to a neurologic problem. Certainly any change in voiding increases the status of the case to an emergency from a routine outpatient encounter. Bowel function is more difficult to evaluate, although fecal incontinence is also an emergency. Pain radiating in a nerve distribution, usually a sciatic distribution down the buttock, along the back of the leg to the back of the knee, down the calf, and then to the posterolateral aspect of the lower leg to the great or small toe, suggests an L5 or S1 nerve entrapment. The pain increases with increased intra-abdominal and intrathoracic pressure and is thus accompanied by coughing, sneezing, and straining for a bowel movement.

Both lumbar strain and HNP occur with trauma and may cause immediately severe pain. Both also radiate, but increased pressure does not increase the radicular component of strain. The history of how posture changes alter pain may be helpful. With HNP, there is usually relief with lying down and flexing hips and knees. Strain does not cause nerve symptoms or signs.

Weakness of a muscle, typically the gastrocnemius or anterior tibialis, always indicates a pinched nerve and should prompt a referral to either a neurologist, neurosurgeon, or orthopedist. Facet syndrome cannot be distinguished from acute strain, although chronic low-grade back pain punctuated by sudden major worsening should suggest a facet or joint etiology.

Numbness is another indication of nerve involvement. Symptoms of numbness, however, are less reliable than signs of numbness as patients experience numbness in a variety of ways. Neurologically significant numbness is present if the patient states that stimulation is perceived less well. Many people will report numbness but will experience no deficit on formal testing. The nature of this symptom is unclear, although it is sometimes the perception of weakness or diminished motor control.

One very important pain syndrome to consider is caused by tumors pressing on the lumbosacral plexus. These are generally slowly progressive and have an insidious onset (unless there is a hemorrhage). The pain is aching or sharp, radiates in a single or multiple nerve distribution, and is unremitting. This pain does not involve the spine, although it may involve the flank or sacroiliac region. Positional changes do not relieve the pain.

Physical Examination

The examination begins with observation for curvature and spasm. Is the lumbar lordosis increased or decreased? Is spasm present? Are any anomalies seen, such as a dimple, that may be associated with spina bifida? Identifying spasm is not usually easy. If the patient is standing, the paraspinal muscles on both sides are normally contracted. I therefore look at the patient while he or she is standing, but palpate the patient while he or she is lying flat, usually supine, placing one hand under the back.

Fasciculations in the legs are rare with most LBP syndromes and are only significant if they accompany wasting and weakness or are seen in only one group of muscles (benign fasciculations are luckily more common than amyotrophic lateral sclerosis). Straight-leg raising will produce back pain if a nerve is compressed, whereas hip flexion with the knee flexed will relieve pressure. Rotating the hip does not worsen nerve root pain. Positive straight-leg raising on the contralateral side supports epidural nerve root compression. A supportive sign of nerve root compression is the recurrence of or increased pain with passive extension of the great toe with the straight-leg raising test.

Strength in each muscle group should be tested but can only be interpreted if pain does not interfere. If a patient gives way because of pain, the examiner can only report that strength was at least that measured when the pain forced the patient to stop. Weakness should not be assumed. Deep tendon reflexes and the sensory examination are important. The history plays a role, however, in the interpretation of the examination. Old back problems, especially operations, may permanently reduce a reflex or sensation. The patient may recall an asymmetry as old, or else a reliable exam from before the injury needs to be obtained. Sensory abnormalities do not always conform to the diagrams in the textbooks, but they should be relatively close. Because the nerve injury is only partial, some parts of the nerve still work and thus the diminished sensation may be patchy. The examiner must be aware of signs that are not physiologic, such as diminished sensation below the knee or groin, because these suggest that, at a minimum, the sensory exam must be considered skeptically or that the entire examination is unreliable.

Gait observation, especially heel and toe walking, may bring out subtle weakness not evident on resistance testing.

Imaging Spine Pain Patients

Although routine spine x-rays are generally not helpful, they should be performed when a malignancy or infection is being considered. Plain spine x-rays are abnormal with metastases to the vertebrae in 85% of cases. For evaluating the typical sprain case, probably only one set of x-rays should be obtained during the first or second episode and not again.

When disk herniation or encroachment on the spinal cord by spondylosis is suspected, or when looking for any lesion pressing on the spinal cord, magnetic resonance imaging (MRI) is the test of choice. For evaluating bone disease, a computed tomography scan is probably better.

TREATMENT OF ACUTE LOW BACK STRAIN

Data on managing patients with LBP are relatively scant and somewhat difficult to interpret because the diagnoses are based on exclusionary rather than inclusionary diagnosis. The options for treatment, however, are quite limited. There is bed rest, limited activity, physical therapy, pain medication, patient education, and chiropractic intervention.

Pain medication is usually restricted to nonsteroidal, anti-inflammatory, and anti–muscle spasm drugs. Narcotics should be restricted to a limited number of doses to prevent dependency.

One study of military recruits found that bed rest produced faster recovery than free ambulation. Another reported that 2 days of bed rest yielded a similar outcome to 7 days of bed rest. However, a third study found that patients whose ambulation was mildly restricted recovered more quickly than those put at bed rest.

Data on physical therapy (PT) are conflicting. Patients are educated, however, during their PT. They learn how to pick up heavy objects and learn exercises that strengthen abdominal muscles, reducing the risk of recurrence. PT is therefore to be encouraged. No data support the use of cold or warm applications, traction, ultrasound, or a transcutaneous electrical nerve stimulator. Chiropractic manipulation may provide some benefits but is considered controversial by most physicians. It is to be avoided in patients with osteoporosis, disk disease, and pinched nerves.

The data on treating acute LBP due to strain and sprain would indicate that, depending on the severity of the pain and the activities and postures that exacerbate it, patients should be advised to avoid activities that aggravate the pain. They should try to maintain ambulatory activities, but if these are too uncomfortable, they should be put at bed rest for up to 2 days. Prolonged bed rest appears to provide no further benefit and increases the problems of deconditioning. It also increases the likelihood of a "sick" role developing, thus initiating a chronic LBP syndrome.

For spasm, carisoprodol, baclofen, and diazepam can be used, but only on a limited basis to avoid inducing depression and pain chronicity.

TREATMENT OF DISK HERNIATION

Although disk herniation is a potentially surgically curable disease, a majority of patients will recover by 6 weeks with only conservative therapy. This consists of bed rest, progressive supervised exercise programs, and education to avoid reinjury. Chiropractic manipulation should be avoided. Some physicians also prescribe prednisone or dexamethasone to reduce inflammation, but these have significant side effects and an uncertain rationale (pinched nerves are not inflamed). This approach should be reserved for the patient who sees a specialist who uses steroids on a regular basis.

TREATMENT OF CHRONIC BACK PAIN

Chronic back pain is perhaps the most difficult clinical problem to manage. These patients come in various categories. There are those with the "failed back syndrome," who have had every operation their doctors recommended yet continue to suffer debilitating pain. There are those whose strain began years before, perhaps in a car accident or in a traumatic incident at work, and despite multiple tests, trials of PT, and education, they continue to suffer. Imaging studies always show arthritis and may show a host of other abnormalities as well.

Most patients with chronic back pain share the same personality profile as other patients with chronic pain, whether it is neck pain, headache, chronic face pain, and so forth.

Each patient requires at least one consultation with a specialist, who must provide a long-term treatment program. Generally this requires settlement of litigation, possible use of antidepressant or chronic pain reducers such as a tricyclics, education about the condition, a graduated exercise program designed for back pain patients, or vocational rehabilitation, if needed. Some patients may respond to occasional injections of steroids into spinal joints, but most require enrollment at behaviorally oriented pain centers. If a chronic back pain treatment center is available, that is the best option, but insurance coverage is often a problem.

THORACIC PAIN

Thoracic pain is far less common than pain in the other spine regions due to reduced flexing and twisting in this region. All the problems that occur in the lumbar spine, however, may occur in the thoracic and must be considered. Metastatic cancer is more common in the thoracic spine than other spine regions and is obviously a serious concern. Cancer pain is usually insidious in onset and gradually progressive because it is initially localized to the involved bone. When the tumor grows outside the bone and causes epidural cord compression, the pain radiates along the involved nerve roots, causing a belt- or girdle-like tightening associated with decreased sensation below.

The major differential diagnostic considerations for thoracic pain with a belt-like sensation or neurologic deficit are thoracic disk herniation and epidural tumors. Tumors are either metastatic, benign spinal canal meningiomas, or lymphomas invading via the foramina from outside the canal. Thoracic disks are uncommon and may present with or without local pain. Unlike lumbar and cervical disks, which can usually be managed conservatively, thoracic disks are usually repaired surgically and generally have good results. These are difficult cases, and surgery should be performed by neurosurgeons with significant experience.

Recurrent thoracic back pain without neurologic symptoms may be managed as LBP is: conservatively, with rest, exercise, and medication, as appropriate. The threshold for radiologic testing should be much lower for thoracic pain than other back pain. Most cases of epidural cord compression from metastatic cancer begin as nonradiating pain localized to one or two vertebrae.

NECK, SHOULDER, AND ARM PAIN

Pain in the neck, like LBP, is a common problem due to multiple etiologies. For some undetermined reason, common parlance ascribes a psychosomatic pain conversion to the neck for some individuals and to a region of the anatomy slightly below the sacrum for others.

The cervical spine consists of seven vertebrae and contains eight nerves. The bones carry significantly less weight than the lower vertebrae but move considerably more, especially the lower cervical ones. The vertebral structure and geometric relationships are the same as the thoracic and the lumbar vertebrae, with the exception of the first two cervical vertebrae, where the dens and the atlas are unique because the C2 vertebra contains the dens (a small extension of the vertebral body that extends upward, providing stabilization for C1). It is the bone fragment that breaks with hanging, getting forced backwards and severing the spinal cord (hangman's fracture).

Pain in the neck and shoulder region is due to problems in the cervical spine, the shoulder itself, or the brachial plexus.

Cervical Spine Pain

Pain from the spine is experienced in the posterior neck, occipital region, shoulder, or arm. The causes of neck pain are similar to those causing lumbar back pain, but their manifestations are somewhat different. In addition, the syndromes of whiplash and thoracic outlet syndromes only occur in the neck.

The most common causes of neck pain are sprain, strain, and arthritis. Unlike LBP, which often is sudden in onset with heavy lifting, neck pain typically arises in a delayed manner or perhaps without an identifiable precipitant.

As in the lower spine, OA is so commonly present on x-ray that the mere finding of OA in an older patient may not be related to the pain. Facet syndromes may cause pain to radiate in a nerve-like distribution but without abnormal neurologic findings on examination. Posterior neck muscles may go into spasm, which are easier to palpitate than spasm in the lower back. These muscles may be tender and frequently limit range of motion.

Disk Disease

Seventy percent of cervical disk herniations involve C7 and 20% involve C6, with C5 and C8 comprising the remaining 10%. Cervical disks tend to herniate posterolaterally, like lumbar disks, but their relationship to the spinal cord is very different. The cervical position of the spinal cord is the fattest part, occupying a significant percentage of the spinal canal, whereas lumbar disks are at a level below the end of the cord. Thus, lumbar disks, if large, can compress multiple roots but not the cord, whereas a large cervical disk may compress a root plus the cord itself.

Disk herniations in the neck may occur after sudden precipitants such as hyperextension, a fall or near fall, or motor vehicle accidents but may also occur without apparent physical stress. A patient may awaken due to neck pain radiating down the course of a nerve (C7 radiates to the middle of the forearm and middle digit and C6 radiates to the thumb and forefinger). There may be objective neurologic signs such as weakness, sensory loss, or a diminished reflex. It can be difficult distinguishing nerve root problems such as carpal tunnel (median nerve) and cubital tunnel (ulnar nerve in the elbow) syndromes from root lesions without accurately charting the distribution of weakness, sensory loss, and deep tendon reflex changes. With minor nerve damage, the clinical signs may be insufficient to judge. Typically, root pain radiates from the neck to the extremity, whereas nerve entrapment pain in the limb radiates from the entrapment proximally, distally, or both.

Spondylosis

Spondylosis is a slowly progressive narrowing of the spinal canal, primarily in the cervical region, due to osteophytic growth around extruded disk material. The pathologic result is often called a "hard disk" to distinguish it from a disk herniation. Cervical spondylosis is a disorder of older patients, whereas disk herniation occurs in the middle-aged. Spondylosis is a slowly progressive problem and appears as ridges on plain cervical spine x-rays. It causes stiffness and pain in the neck, shoulder, and arm and causes focal spine problems (see Chapter 5, Gait Disorders). The ridges may compress cervical roots, causing radicular arm pain and neuropathic symptoms, but, most important, compression of the cord may cause bladder dysfunction (urgency and frequency from "spastic" bladder) or spastic gait.

Arthritis

Although related to spondylosis, arthritic changes are restricted to the joints. As in the lumbar spine, these may cause a facet pain syndrome that radiates down the arm but without neurologic signs, or may compress roots in the neural foramen, like growths of stalagmites or stalactites in caves. In the latter case, neurologic signs are frequently present. Neuropathic signs and symptoms, as well as arthritic pain, are often exacerbated by pressing down on the patient's head during the neurologic exam, especially when the head is turned. Pulling up on the head may relieve tension in the foramen and thus reduce symptoms.

Strain and Sprain

As with LBP, *strain* and *sprain* are the terms we apply to all patients with neck pain who have no neurologic signs but who have muscle pain. This often occurs after prolonged strained neck postures such as craning one's neck to paint the ceiling or to tile a floor. Using a pillow of the wrong height to sleep at night may produce chronic neck pain.

Whiplash

Whiplash is the term applied to the sudden acceleration and deceleration that occurs in a car accident. The head is suddenly thrown in one direction and then back again. The pain starts 1 or 2 days after the injury and is muscular in nature. Its duration depends on the force of the impact and often on the presence of litigation.

More than 1 million Americans suffer whiplash injuries each year. Twenty to forty percent have symptoms lasting for years. While many of these cases may be related to legal and financial issues, many injuries persist despite the absence of pending litigation or other obvious secondary gain. A controlled trial of steroid injections to facet joints to relieve whiplash pain was not helpful and is therefore not recommended. Definitive treatment does not exist. Acute injury should be treated with analgesics, and a soft collar, if used, should not be used more than a few days.

Brachial Plexus

Lesions of the brachial plexus are rare. They fall into three categories: tumor, trauma, and an idiopathic entity called *brachial neuritis*. Tumors involving the brachial plexus are usually apical lung tumors, although infiltrating lymphomas can cause the same problem. Brachial neuralgia is indistinguishable from this clinically. The patient develops unremitting aching pain in the shoulder girdle with clear focal neurologic signs. Atrophy and fasciculations are seen if the syndrome has been present for a few weeks.

Traumatic injuries are either due to direct crush injuries or to hyperextension injuries of the head or an arm, causing severe traction on the nerves. While the symptoms are the same as the tumor and neuritis syndromes, the history clearly separates the syndromes.

Management

Neck pain with neurologic signs requires an MRI of the cervical spine and a referral to a neurologist or neurosurgeon. Myelopathy, manifest by gait spasticity, is probably the most urgent of these problems. Neck pain with nerve root symptoms but without signs probably requires an MRI and possibly an electromyogram (EMG). Neck pain without neurologic signs is generally best managed with a soft collar, nonsteroidal anti-inflammatory drugs, and reassurance. Sustained pain without recovery should prompt referral to an orthopedist or rheumatologist. In general, patients should be warned against participating in any activity that worsens the pain. PT may be started after the acute pain remits. If the pain becomes chronic, referral to a behavioral medicine pain clinic should be considered.

Chiropractic manipulation, while often useful for the low back, is considered potentially dangerous for neck problems, and most neurologists caution against this.

CLINICAL PEARLS

- Cervical radiculopathies involve C7 70% of the time, C6 20% of the time, and C5 or C8 the remaining 10% of the time.
- Cervical disk herniation may cause spinal cord problems.
- Lumbar disk herniation occurs below the terminus of the spinal cord and can only cause lower motor neuron problems.
- Thoracic spine pain should raise a suspicion of metastatic cancer.
- Prolonged bed rest is no better than 2 days of bed rest for acute lumbar strain.
- Chronic neck and lower back pain are exceedingly difficult management problems for which there is no single best approach.
- Litigation complicates treatment of all spine pain problems.
- Increasing leg weakness and numbness with walking downhill suggest a diagnosis of spinal stenosis, not spinal cord or leg claudication.
- Coughing, sneezing, and straining for a bowel movement frequently reproduce neuropathic symptoms when there is epidural nerve compression.
- Lying flat with the knees flexed usually relieves back pain from an HNP.
- Thoracic outlet syndrome is an exceedingly rare disorder requiring EMG confirmation for diagnosis.

4

Epilepsy, Fainting, and Episodic Disorders

Seizure and *epilepsy* are not synonymous terms. *Epilepsy* is the name reserved for the syndrome of two or more unprovoked seizures. Repeated seizures from hypoglycemia, alcohol withdrawal, or other known seizure precipitants are not considered epilepsy. Epilepsy is a common disorder, third in frequency among neurologic problems in American adults. By the age of 80, more than 10% of Americans have had a seizure at some time, and 0.5–1.0% have epilepsy. The incidence, meaning the new development of epilepsy, is high in prepubescent children, drops and remains low in young and middle-age adults, and then increases with age after age 60, presumably due to strokes, Alzheimer's disease, intracranial neoplasms, and trauma.

It is important to understand what a seizure is, yet defining *seizure* is not straightforward. There are convulsive and nonconvulsive seizures, pseudoseizures, fugue states, behavioral dyscontrol syndromes, and various other brief behavioral alterations that may be difficult to distinguish from each other. A seizure is a transient alteration in behavior caused by an uncontrolled, abnormally synchronous discharge of cortical neurons. The feature that distinguishes a seizure from other transient disorders is the electrical discharge in the cortex of the brain.

Seizures may be inherited, symptomatic, or idiopathic and may be precipitated or unprovoked. Repeated seizures due to hypoxia, hypoglycemia, hyponatremia, alcohol withdrawal, or a host of other disorders are not indicative of epilepsy. Repeated seizures due to cortical scars from stroke, traumatic injury, central nervous system infection, or other static pathology are called *symptomatic epilepsy*. Virtually all adult acquired epilepsy is thought to be symptomatic in the sense that a cortical injury is the presumed etiology, but in many cases, if not most, the etiology cannot be identified and the syndrome is labeled *idiopathic epilepsy*. Inherited epilepsies are uncommon. Adult acquired epilepsy is generally thought to be the result of old head trauma or stroke. Tumors, particularly meningiomas, are relatively common in the elderly and cause a substantial minority of epileptic syndromes. Small arteriovenous malformations, brain maldevelopments, and other structural abnormalities are rare.

Epileptic seizures have been classified by the International League Against Epilepsy based on clinical and electroencephalogram (EEG) characteristics into four major groups: partial seizures, generalized seizures, status epilepticus, and unclassified seizures (Table 4.1). Partial seizures have a focal onset that may be seen clinically, perhaps with the eyes deviating to one side or one arm stiffening or shaking first, or on the EEG with a focal onset, even when the clinical manifestations appear to affect both sides simultaneously without any asymmetry. Partial seizures are divided into three subcategories: simple, with no alteration of consciousness; complex partial, with altered consciousness but no frank loss of consciousness; and secondary generalized, which begin at one location and spread to cause a generalized convulsion. Generalized seizures affect the whole body simultaneously and originate on both sides of the brain simultaneously. Status epilepticus is defined by continuous seizures or recurrent seizures without a return to consciousness. The patient who recovers after a seizure and then has another seizure can be described as having a flurry of seizures, whereas the term *status epilepticus* carries a degree of seriousness and possible ominous outcome that the term *flurry* does not.

Generalized seizures are almost always convulsive in adults and involve loss of consciousness. Nonconvulsive seizures, such as atonic seizures or petit mal absence seizures, are rarely encountered by the

Table 4.1.   Epilepsy classification

I. Partial (onset is focal)
  A. Simple (no impairment of consciousness)
    1. Motor-stiffening or jerking (may affect one side synchro-
       nously or may march up or down)
    2. Sensory (abnormal sensation and no external concomitant)
    3. Autonomic (major disturbance with diaphoresis, diarrhea,
       tachycardia)
  B. Complex partial (impaired consciousness with automatisms)
  C. Secondarily generalized (focal onset [by electroencephalogram
     (EEG) or observation] followed by generalized motor activity)
II. Generalized (EEG-confirmed onset over entire cortex)
  A. Petit mal (childhood onset)
  B. Tonic, clonic, tonic/clonic
  C. Atonic
III. Other (rare)
IV. Status epilepticus

primary care physician (PCP) treating adults. Nonconvulsive
seizures such as petit mal, described below, involve brief lapses of
attention with minor or no motor concomitant. Atonic seizures, in
which patients simply lose tone and drop, as in a sudden faint, only
occur in patients who also have other forms of epilepsy that tend to
be poorly controlled.

PHENOMENOLOGY

Most witnessed seizures are easy to identify. The spells that are difficult to classify are, fortunately, uncommon, even for neurologists.
Most seizures are generalized, meaning that they involve the whole
cortex and are usually manifest as grand mal ("big bad") seizures.
The patient suffering a seizure usually loses consciousness suddenly,
while simultaneously stiffening, entering the tonic or stiff part of the
seizure. The patient may make a sound due to air suddenly being
expelled as the chest muscles tighten. This is the epileptic cry. This
phase lasts a few seconds and is followed by partial relaxation,

repeated tonic contractions, or clonic contractions. Tonic contractions induce a posture that is sustained for seconds at a time, whereas clonic movements are gross muscle jerks. The clonic phase of a seizure typically follows a tonic phase and may be sandwiched between two tonic phases. During the tonic phase the patient frequently becomes cyanotic from extraordinary muscular effort without breathing. Although frightening to observe, this is not a cause for concern in most patients. Incontinence is common in seizures and may occur during the muscle contraction or at the end, during relaxation. Most patients are comatose immediately after a seizure and return to a normal mental state over several minutes to hours. On awakening there is be a period of confusion that slowly resolves. Headache, severe muscle aches, and profound sleepiness are common sequelae. A transient low-grade fever is also common.

Complex partial seizures are spells in which consciousness is altered but not lost. Memory for the period of the event is impaired. These are frequently called *temporal lobe seizures* or *petit mal*, but both terms are incorrect and should be discouraged. Petit mal refers to a specific seizure disorder of children (discussed below) that rarely presents in adults. Since the nature, pathophysiology, prognosis, and treatment of the petit mal seizure are different than those of temporal lobe or complex partial seizures, the term *petit mal* should be restricted to its appropriate use. Although most complex partial seizures are in fact of temporal lobe origin, about 20–25% are not, making the term *temporal lobe seizure* inaccurate. Its use, however, does not create problems. During a complex partial seizure the patient suddenly tunes out, looks interested in something not there or stares blankly, and generally performs meaningless automatic movements like blinking, lip smacking, face rubbing, or dial turning. The person may respond to verbal queries but always abnormally, as if intoxicated or hearing the voice through a dense fog. Physical intervention, such as restraining, may induce a defensive response and lead to a scuffle. One of my patients starts climbing on tables or chairs during her seizures and needs to be held back to avoid injury. Another simply stares off suddenly and raises his arms, keeping them in place as if prepared to ward off an attack. Another stares fearfully, pats her face, and picks her nose. After these spells, the patient is confused and usually, but not always, realizes that a seizure has occurred. During complex partial spells, patients may be incontinent. There are reports in the epilepsy literature of patients having long periods of amnesia during which they competently performed complex acts. Stories of doctors accurately diagnosing and treating medical problems while having complex partial seizures or performing operations have been published. I am highly skeptical and suspect that most, if not all, such spells were of psychiatric origin. Seizures of frontal lobe origin produce the most bizarre behaviors, including gelastic (laughing) seizures, masturbatory seizures, and other markedly abnormal behaviors. Like complex partial seizures of temporal lobe origin, they usually last half a minute to 2 minutes and are followed by a postictal state. These patients are frequently misdiagnosed as having a psychiatric disorder.

Simple partial seizures are those without a change in mental state. Simple motor seizures involve involuntary movements, which may be tonic or clonic. The famous "jacksonian march" of Hughlings Jackson describes a seizure beginning in one spot of the motor cortex, manifest by thumb twitches, then traveling up the cortex, simultaneously "marching" up the arm, then spreading to the leg. Simple seizures are invariably unilateral. If they spread to the other side, consciousness is impaired. I once consulted on a case allegedly involving seizurelike movements on both sides without impaired consciousness. The patient actually had involuntary movements on one side. She was bothered by the movements, however, and tried to contain them by using her good arm and good leg to prevent the involved side from moving. To the (obviously) untrained intern, this was a bilateral seizure. Simple sensory seizures, like motor seizures, are limited to one side and usually involve an abnormal, uncomfortable sensation. It is generally the case that seizure phenomena represent positive phenomena (a movement, a burning or tingling sensation, or a hallucination), in contrast to ischemic events, which usually produce negative phenomena, weakness, paralysis, sensations of deadness or numbness, and so on. Other simple seizures, though quite rare, are autonomic seizures, which are accompanied by brief spells of profound diaphoresis, blood pressure elevation, tachycardia, or diarrhea, or special sensory seizures that are accompanied by visual hallucinations of usually simple geometric shapes or colors.

Petit mal seizures are childhood-onset seizures that begin between the ages of 4 and 12. They almost always either resolve during puberty or are transformed into generalized seizures. These spells are brief, typically lasting less than 20 seconds, during which the child simply stares ahead as if in a trance. The EEG is diagnostic, showing three-per-second generalized spike and wave complexes in every channel. The spells only occur while the child is sedentary, so they draw little or no attention other than for a decline in school performance, because there may be hundreds or even thousands of seizures daily. The child is unaware of the seizures. Teachers see the child "daydreaming" or not paying attention. Because the attacks are unknown to the child, he or she may lose seconds of every minute's worth of conversation. School starts to become more difficult. When seizures last several seconds, there may be eye blinking or lip smacking at the rate of three per second. These spells look exactly like complex partial seizures but have no postictal confusion.

Febrile seizures are a childhood syndrome, generally limited to children between 6 months and 5 years of age. With high fevers from any source the child experiences a generalized convulsion. These last longer than seizures in adults, sometimes more than 20 minutes. There are no sequelae to uncomplicated febrile seizures, which are those that lack focality and last less than 30 minutes. They are not usually treated, but, if they are, aggressively lowering the body temperature is the treatment of choice. Adults with seizures and high fevers are presumed to have a central nervous system infection or aspiration pneumonia, not febrile seizures.

A rare but interesting epileptic syndrome called *reflex epilepsy* may be mislabeled as psychogenic. In reflex epilepsy, particular stimuli produce a reflex convulsion. The most common stimulus is flashing lights, but cases have been documented in which particular pieces of music, even particular songs sung by one singer, produce a seizure. Such a case was used as the basis for an episode of the TV show *Seinfeld*.

NONEPILEPTIC SPELLS

Pseudoseizures are spells that look like epileptic seizures but have a psychiatric or malingering origin. Some spells are easily diagnosed because they occur at times of stress, last unusually long periods of time, and can display obviously symbolic behavior. These spells, like all episodic psychiatric disorders, can be divided into those that are due to malingering and those that are presumably unconscious. The former are probably easier to diagnose, occurring for clear gain, whereas the latter represent a conversion disorder and are precipitated by psychic stressors that are not clear to the patient. The spells may look like atypical grand mal or complex partial seizures. Whereas these spells, if witnessed (which is not usually the case), may be diagnosed appropriately, a study using videotaped organic and pseudoseizures determined that epilepsy experts could not do better than chance in distinguishing peculiar (generally frontal lobe) complex partial seizures from pseudoseizures. Thus, even witnessing a spell may not allow diagnosis. Organic seizures, both grand mal and complex partial, produce an immediate, very large increase in the serum prolactin level so that a blood specimen should be obtained immediately after a possible pseudoseizure, if it occurs while in the emergency room (ER) or the office, for diagnostic purposes. An EEG during a spell would be better. A marked elevation confirms the diagnosis. A normal level does not exclude the diagnosis but makes it less likely. When observing a spell suspected of being psychogenic or malingering it may be helpful both for diagnosis and for treatment to suggest a behavior that can stop the attack. Statements ostensibly to a nurse but really for the patient's benefit, such as "If this is really a seizure, it should end in 15 seconds," or "Once I apply pressure to the eyes the seizure will stop, if it's real," may be useful. Some physicians announce threats, such as "If it doesn't stop soon I'll have to give that really painful medicine" or something similar. If one uses suggestions, it should always be to help the situation, not worsen it. Never suggest a new symptom. I believe that pseudoseizures, unless clearly malingering in nature, should always be evaluated by a neurologist. The nature of these spells is that they frequently go hand-in-hand with organic seizures, so that the unfortunate patient suffers from both. Most patients with presumed pseudoseizures should be evaluated with prolonged (8- to 36-hour) continuous EEG with closed circuit videotape monitoring in the hope of capturing a spell and correlating the EEG with the videotaped behavior.

Other spells that may be misdiagnosed as seizures are as uncommon as they are interesting. These poorly understood spells include paroxysmal movement disorders (ataxia, dystonia, and chorea) and paroxysmal sleep disorders. The paroxysmal movement disorders are often inherited and typically begin in childhood. Most spells last hours, but some may be much shorter. There is no mental impairment, and the movements are either ataxic, dystonic, or choreic and do not usually look like seizure-induced movements such as tonic extension, clonus, or automatisms. Sleep disorders include periodic leg movements during sleep, which are usually isolated leg jerks, sometimes in flurries but not occurring in a sustained fashion, and rapid eye movement (REM) behavior disorder. The latter is almost always associated with parkinsonism (sometimes predating its development) and is a syndrome of older men in which the patient, who should be paralyzed during the dream (REM) phase of sleep, is not, so that the patient acts out the dream, invariably dreams of running and fighting. These occur infrequently and often cause injuries, either to the patient from jumping out of bed into the wall or to the spouse from being choked or beaten. The patient does this during sleep and on awakening cannot recall the episode, although sometimes can recall the dream. These may be misdiagnosed as complex partial seizures.

Episodic dyscontrol syndromes in which patients suddenly become belligerent are sometimes confused with epilepsy because patients are sometimes amnestic for the incident. However, the history invariably confirms a preceding period of building rage that was waiting for a trigger, no matter how minor. The attacks are frequently stereotyped and are always an attack on a particular person (step-father, mother, sister, or other close acquaintance), and the patient often feels remorse afterward. During the spell, the patient is out of control from rage, not delirium. Micro-sleeps are sudden sleep attacks occurring in sleep-deprived individuals who tend to fall asleep while driving. They awaken without recollection of the event and may not recall feeling sleepy. Convulsive syncope is discussed in the section on faints.

Fugue states are prolonged periods lasting hours to days during which the subject acts normally but is later amnestic for the entire spell. Patients cannot recall their names, their parents, their date of birth, and so forth. Transient global amnesia is a very stereotypical syndrome of unknown etiology in which a patient, usually middle-aged or elderly but sometimes younger, suddenly becomes amnestic for a period of several hours. During this period they ask the same questions over and over again and are often mildly distressed. Old memories of cognitive function are intact, so they appear to have a Korsakoff's psychosis but with the added feature of repetitive questioning.

Evaluation

Most seizures are evaluated in the ER. If the patient is a known epileptic, the ER visit is usually not beneficial to the patient. Frequently when a seizure occurs at work or in a public setting, an ambulance is called and the patient, postictal, cannot explain to the rescue workers that an ER trip is not required. If the patient is not a known epileptic, then all the different etiologies for seizures must be considered. These are structural, metabolic, toxic, infectious, and traumatic.

In the ER the patient is stabilized and blood is sent for glucose, sodium, calcium, blood urea nitrogen, magnesium, anticonvulsants, and toxicology evaluations. If the patient is seizing or not lightening up, thiamine and an ampule of D50 is given (if the patient is hypoglycemic, this is helpful, and if he or she is hyperglycemic it does not matter). If the patient is not actively seizing, there is no need for either diazepam or lorazepam. These drugs, which prolong the postictal stuporous state, should be reserved for stopping active seizures only.

For patients who have had their first seizure, a brain image is the most important initial test, once blood work reveals no metabolic explanation. The computed tomography (CT) scan or magnetic resonance imaging (MRI) must exclude stroke, tumor, and brain trauma or abscess. Even when a metabolic explanation is found, a brain CT scan should be performed to explore the possibility that a focal lesion was present and the seizure threshold was lowered by the metabolic derangement. In the ER, the CT scan usually is done without contrast either because it is obtained on an emergency basis and squeezed into the schedule or is obtained at night without a radiologist present to inject the dye. If an MRI is obtained, a CT scan is unnecessary. MRI is preferable to a CT scan because it is less likely to miss small cortical lesions. In patients without a clear metabolic explanation for their seizure, an MRI should be obtained.

What may surprise non-neurologists is the question of whether an EEG should be performed. A person with a normal CT scan and a clear-cut metabolic explanation for the seizures should have one EEG, but a patient with recurrent provoked spells should not have it repeated. The person with an unprovoked first seizure should have an EEG to assess risk of further recurrence because not all unprovoked first seizures require treatment. Certain abnormal EEG patterns may dictate choice of drug or even prognosis.

Patients with recurrent spells of uncertain type should have an EEG. When the EEG is nondiagnostic and seizures are still suspected, longer EEG monitoring is indicated. Although 24-hour ambulatory EEGs are commercially available, prolonged closed circuit video EEGs are preferable. They are less contaminated by artifact and reveal the behavioral alterations in synchrony with the EEG.

Treatment

When to treat is the first question. Over the last 10 years there has been a huge change in our approach to seizure management. Until the 1980s, most physicians would prescribe an anticonvulsant drug (ACD) for any unprovoked seizure. Further seizures occurring on one ACD would produce a prescription for a second and then a third ACD, resulting in a patient more debilitated by drug toxicity than by seizures. Finally, few doctors stopped an ACD once begun, no matter how long the patient had been seizure free. With more data to answer the most obvious but previously unasked questions, our approaches to these three core issues have changed.

Only about one-third of patients with a first unprovoked seizure suffer a second spell within 5 years. Thus, patients who have a first unprovoked seizure should be told that they are unlikely to have another seizure but are at greater risk than "normal" people. Most patients prefer to take their 33% risk rather than take medicine regularly and possibly be labeled by their health insurer or employer as epileptic. On the other hand, some patients report that their seizure was so unpleasant or the risk is so unacceptable that they would rather take medication and have their ACD levels checked by regular blood testing to reduce their seizure risk as much as possible. Thus, the decision to treat or not needs to be adequately discussed. The risk of further seizures increases with an abnormal neurologic exam or an abnormal EEG, so these should be factored into decision making. An EEG showing an active epileptiform focus should sway the decision toward treatment.

Two unprovoked seizures occurring within a couple of years of each other indicate a need for an ACD. This is a clinical decision independent of the EEG. If the first seizure was adequately evaluated with a brain imaging study and an EEG, a repeat EEG is probably not needed.

Forty to fifty percent of epileptic patients can be maintained seizure free on a single ACD. What medication should be used? For grand mal seizures, whether primarily or secondarily generalized, and for complex partial seizures the drugs of choices are the four "old line" drugs: phenytoin, phenobarbital, carbamazepine, and valproic acid. Now that carbamazepine comes in a long-acting form, all of these drugs can be given twice daily. The enormous improvement in compliance that accompanies bid versus tid or qid dosing results in dramatically improved seizure control. Phenytoin (Dilantin) and valproate (Depakote) are easiest to start because they are relatively nonsedating. Phenytoin can be loaded orally by giving two doses of 500 mg a few hours apart. This may cause ataxia, but is usually well tolerated. The patient should then be given 300 mg (5 mg/kg/day) daily, 200 mg at night and 100 mg in the morning. A serum level can be checked after 4–6 days. Increases in dosing should be made cautiously, because phenytoin kinetics are such that serum levels go up slowly until albumin binding is complete, then rise rapidly (along with toxicity). Thus, the phenytoin level may rise a small amount with the first increase of 100 mg but then rise dramatically with the next increase. Since phenytoin may cause hirsutism, gingival hyperplasia, and the fetal hydantoin syndrome, it is not a good drug for girls and young women. Valproic acid is generally well tolerated but is not usually given as a loading dose. It should be started at 15 mg/kg/day in two divided doses of Depakote and increased by 5–10 mg/kg/day each week (250–500 mg/day). If it needs to be started quickly, the short-acting formulation, valproic acid (Depakene), should be given in 500-mg oral boluses on a q6h regimen, then switched to Depakote, 500 mg q12h.

Phenobarbital has been the drug of choice for a woman who wants to conceive because more data about its fetal effects are available about it than for any other ACD. There is a question, however, of whether phenobarbital may lead to mild intellectual impairment in the fetus and whether it may also lead to a bleeding disorder in the newborn. Pregnant women should receive vitamin K to prevent bleeding disorders. Phenobarbital is, of course, quite sedating for the first few weeks. Carbamazepine (Tegretol XR) needs to be started at a low dose and increased slowly. Generally a higher dose may be given in the evening, starting at 200 mg at night and 100 mg in the morning, increasing as tolerated (every 3–5 days) to about 300 mg q12h while monitoring the ACD level. With phenytoin and phenobarbital, no blood work other than measurement of the ACD level is required. This should be checked every 2–4 weeks until stable. With carbamazepine, the serum should be checked every 3 weeks until stable. A white blood cell count needs to be checked after about 4 weeks. The occurrence of aplastic anemia or agranulocytosis from carbamazepine is very rare and appears to be irreversible so that routine monitoring of the blood count is more grounded in tradition than common sense. With valproate, liver function tests need to be checked in children. The ACD should be checked weekly until stable. Once the serum ACD level is in the therapeutic range and stable and if the patient is tolerating the drug, the dose should be maintained. When new medications are begun or old medications are stopped, their effects on the ACD level should be researched and, in cases of interactions, the level needs to be rechecked. All ACD levels should be checked at their low point, or trough level, to assess the point of least protection.

In patients first starting an ACD, the level should be checked every 3 months or so once stable and then every 6 months after two or three checks are acceptable. In cases in which seizures are well controlled but ACD levels are consistently low (but measurable) or high without toxicity, I recommend not adjusting the medication. It is important to keep in mind that the therapeutic level is a target that represents a statistically derived range and is not necessarily ideal for any particular individual.

Patients whose seizures are not adequately controlled with one medication should be referred to a neurologist. In general, a neurologist should push the first drug to a higher level, then switch to a different first-line medication, get it into the therapeutic range, and then stop the first. It is always best to aim for single drug treatment over polypharmacy to avoid adverse effects. Only 10% of patients inadequately controlled on a single ACD are controlled on two or more drugs. Thus, three drugs are rarely a wise choice. It is also wise to aim to use old drugs with known side effects in preference to any of the newer ACDs—gabapentin, lamotrigine, or topiramide. Although a common practice in the past, there is no reason to obtain annual EEGs in epileptics. Once the decision is made to use an ACD, further EEGs are indicated only if seizures worsen or if decisions concerning ACD discontinuation or epilepsy surgery are being made.

Stopping Anticonvulsants

Patients who have had few seizures, have been seizure free for 2–4 years on a single ACD, and who have a normal neurologic exam and a normal EEG can have their ACD tapered slowly and stopped. The patient must agree to the decision, of course, knowing that the risk of a repeat seizure, while small, is not nil. The impact of a repeat seizure while driving needs to be considered. The taper should be over 1–3 months, depending on the drug dose. It is usually wise to have a neurologist's help to make this decision. An abnormal EEG due to nonepileptiform problems is cause for concern but is not an absolute contraindication to drug discontinuation, just as an abnormal neurologic exam is not. Epileptiform activity on the EEG, however, should abort ACD stoppage.

QUALITY OF LIFE

The quality-of-life issues in epilepsy are important and usually center on the safety of driving. All states have driving restrictions on epileptics, although none restricts insulin-dependent diabetics or patients with cardiac arrhythmias. Most states require a seizure-free period of half a year to 1 year before allowing an epileptic to drive. The same is true for a patient with a single unprovoked seizure. If a seizure occurs during an attempt to stop the ACD, then a more brief period of not driving is required in some states once the patient is back on the ACD.

FITS, FAINTS, AND FALLS

Unwitnessed spells of lost consciousness are a common problem, particularly in the elderly. If the person's walking and balance are normal, the differential is between seizures and syncope. With impaired gait or balance, one must also include trips and falls. For most falls and faints, the history is diagnostic, whether the spell was observed or not. If the patient struck his or her head, however, then there may have been a concussion, inducing brief retrograde amnesia that prevents any recollection of the event.

Vasovagal syncope is usually preceded by a fairly stereotypical presyncopal experience. The patient feels lightheaded, tired, possibly nauseated, and diaphoretic and feels everything becoming distant or dark. The next thing he knows, he is waking up on the floor. Body tone is lost, so the fall is fairly soft and injuries are less common than in seizures. A witness may observe the body collapsing "like a sack of potatoes." Recovery usually occurs within seconds of lying supine, and unless there is head trauma, the patient is back to normal on awakening, other than for the confusion of sorting out what just took place. The patient may feel refreshed but not fatigued, achy, or have a headache. Some people, on fainting, have a few myoclonic or clonic jerks and tonic posturing, and may be incontinent of urine. However, they manifest no postictal confusional state, and the convulsive aspect lasts only a few seconds. These episodes, with a brief convulsive episode, are very hard to distinguish from a seizure unless witnessed by the physician or accompanied by a history that strongly implicates a faint (e.g., presyncopal symptoms or a cardiac arrhythmia). This syndrome is called *convulsive syncopy*. Faints occur while the patient is standing and occasionally while seated, but not while lying supine, whereas seizures are independent of posture as they are unrelated to blood pressure. If a grand mal seizure occurs with the person standing or walking, the patient stiffens and topples like a board. The powerful muscle contractions may cause posterior shoulder displacements or tongue macerations from the molars' clamping down.

Cardiac syncope may cause sudden syncope with few or no premonitory symptoms. Finally, transient ischemic attacks do not cause loss of consciousness without causing other brain stem dysfunction. Thus, vertebrobasilar insufficiency (VBI) is unlikely without symptoms of diplopia, ataxia, hemiparesis, or true vertigo. In cases of unwitnessed loss of consciousness with concussion, VBI must also be considered.

Unwitnessed spells of lost consciousness, especially in the elderly when a history is unavailable, are statistically far more likely to represent syncope or a fall than anything else. The evaluation should be oriented in that direction. The physical examination should focus on the heart, with an extended evaluation of the heart rate, and must also include measurement of orthostatic blood pressure changes. Gait and balance must be observed to assess the possibility of a fall. EEG is the diagnostic study of choice for seizures but is often normal or nonspecifically abnormal in the evaluation of a seizure. It is less useful for diagnosis than for localization (e.g., surgery).

CLINICAL PEARLS

- Ischemia usually causes "negative" phenomena, whereas seizures generally cause "positive" phenomena. Thus, strokes usually cause weakness or numbness (a "dead" or "wooden" sensation). Seizures typically cause jerking, stiffness, tingling, burning, or other uncomfortable sensations.
- Syncope usually does not result in injuries. People tend to fall relatively gently. Seizures are much more likely to cause injuries as the subject falls while either rigid (tonic phase) or jerking (clonic phase). Shoulder injuries such as subluxation and humeral fracture that occur during unwitnessed spells of lost consciousness are highly suggestive of seizures and not fainting spells.
- Alcohol withdrawal seizures are generalized and nonfocal and usually occur in flurries about 12–36 hours after the last drink.
- Seventy percent of epileptics are maintained seizure free on one anticonvulsant drug.
- Only 10% of patients who continue to have seizures on adequate trials of a single anticonvulsant drug achieve control on two-drug therapy.
- Dizziness is rarely of neurologic origin.
- A low serum anticonvulsant level should be interpreted as meaning the patient takes his or her medication. Look for high metabolic rate or drug interaction before assuming noncompliance.

- Most anticonvulsants reduce the efficacy of birth control pills.
- Most organic seizures transiently increase serum prolactin levels, whereas most pseudoseizures do not. Therefore a prolactin level in a recently postictal patient may help distinguish organic and pseudoseizures.
- Seizures of frontal lobe onset may produce extremely bizarre behavior that appears to be psychiatric.
- All presumed pseudoseizure patients should be evaluated by a neurologist.
- Abnormal behavior patterns lasting more than 5 minutes (for the seizure plus the postictal state to improve) should raise a concern for a psychiatric explanation. A history of childhood sexual and physical abuse should be explored.

5

Gait Disorders

Gait disorders become increasingly common with agir.g. Falls constitute the single most common cause of traumatic death and injury in elderly Americans. There are more than 200,000 hip fractures yearly from falls in the United States. In addition to falls, impaired walking may cause disability, and fear of falling may itself initiate a gait problem. Although most gait abnormalities are not of neurologic origin, a high percentage are. The impact of gait disturbances is so great and so many falls are preventable that more attention should be paid to walking and balance problems in the primary care setting. All abnormalities of gait require explanation, even in the elderly. This does not mean, of course, that all patients need to be seen by a specialist. It does mean that the primary care physician should have a good explanation as to why the patient needs a cane or walker or why there are occasional falls. It is common for patients to be examined without having their walking observed. The patient is placed in an examining room and is visited by the physician. When the physician is finished with the general examination, he or she moves on to the next patient. On numerous occasions, I have evaluated patients admitted to the hospital because of falls or walking problems whose actual walking has never before been examined. Such a consult request might read, "Evaluate for leg weakness. Patient unable to walk." More often than not, the legs are not weak and the patient has Parkinson's disease or a spastic paraparesis.

Usually the reason the patient walks abnormally or requires an assistive device is ascertained by simply asking the patient. The most common etiologies are musculoskeletal problems such as arthritis or bunions. Visual loss complicates the problem. It is not infrequent, however, that the patient does not know why he or she is walking poorly. In these situations the physician must determine a reasonable explanation.

FAINTS, FALLS, AND TRIPS

Before approaching the topic of gait dysfunction, I think it reasonable to discuss falling. The term *fall* actually has a technical meaning. The Kellogg International Working Group defined *fall* as "an event which results in a person coming to rest inadvertently on the ground or other lower level and other than as a consequence of the following: sustaining a violent blow; loss of consciousness; sudden onset of paralysis as in a stroke; or an epileptic seizure." It is important to distinguish a fall from a trip and from a faint when possible. When the event is unwitnessed, however, and the patient ended up on the ground and has hit his or her head, this may be impossible. Using common sense, one can determine that a trip occurs when the environment somehow intrudes on the person's walking. A foot catches the leg of a table, a rug slips, a patch of ice is encountered, a crack in the cement is not noticed, and so forth. Balance is lost, and the person lands on the ground. A faint is the loss of consciousness without preceding head trauma. Most occur with the patient upright and are preceded by an aura of lightheadedness, nausea, diaphoresis, sleepiness, a sensation of the room becoming "distant," or having vision fade, followed by awakening on the floor. Most faints do not result in injuries, as the patient gradually loses body tone and falls "like a sack of potatoes." This is unlike a trip, where the patient is moving when the foot catches, or slips, causing the person to be propelled toward the ground. In any case, however, if the head strikes any object, there is, in addition to the surprise of the event, a possible concussion with brief loss of memory for the time before the episode. Faints require a cardiovascular evaluation and are rarely of neurologic origin (see Chapter 4). Trips are considered a routine hazard of everyday life but rarely cause falls for normal people. Falls, however, are always patho-logic. A fall is an event in which the person hits the ground for no environmental reason. It is due to a problem with maintaining bal-ance. Inner ear dysfunction with associated vertigo may cause falls. Parkinson's disease and related conditions may cause patients to catch their feet on the floor, or to freeze suddenly and be unable to move their feet as they are moving forward, or to spontaneously fall backward when standing in one spot. Cerebellar and sensory ataxias (discussed later) also cause loss of balance, similar to intoxications due to the brain's inability to keep the center of gravity properly maintained. Posterior spinal cord disorders cause loss of position sense and, hence, a sensory ataxia. Spasticity causes abnormal leg con-trol so that although the sense of balance is normal, the legs may not be able to achieve stability. Balance problems may be due to prob-lems of information input, information output, or sensory-motor inte-gration in the various gait centers of the brain.

To interpret gait abnormalities, one should understand normal gait as a touchstone. Clinical gait analysis—that is, the interpretation of gait abnormalities by visual inspection—is remarkably compli-cated. Laboratories study both the normal and pathologic gait using a variety of sophisticated measures of muscle contractions and dis-tances moved by various joints and their responses to perturbations. Most clinical gait laboratories are devoted to the analysis of gait in children with cerebral palsy to determine what orthopedic surgical maneuvers might best help the child walk better.

How one performs a simple visual analysis of gait depends on one's background and sensitivity to the problem. Podiatrists, orthopedists, and neurologists tend to look at gait from remarkably different per-spectives. Podiatrists obviously focus on the feet, looking for varus and valgus orientations, heel strike, foot rotation, and deformities. Ortho-pedists tend to look for joint problems, particularly at the knees and hips, and therefore at asymmetries of gait; for scoliosis, indicating leg length differences; and spasticity, particularly in children. Neurologists focus more on posture, balance, and arm swing. An interesting example of the different perspectives is in a well-written introductory book on gait analysis that fails to discuss posture and arm swing at all. It even shows a "normal" gait cycle without arm movements. This occurred because arm swing is not important for the biomechanics of walking, playing virtually no role in the energy requirements or coordination of normal walking. To a neurologist, however, it may be an extremely important clinical sign, especially when asymmetric. Although arm swing is not important for walking, it may be a crucial sign for the diagnosis of Parkinson's disease, brain tumor, or other serious disorders.

A complicating feature of gait analysis, as is true in so much of medicine and particularly neurology, is the gray area of what distinguishes normal from pathologic in the elderly. We all can look at the trim and fit 80-year-old who participates in the Senior Olympics and agree he looks remarkably healthy. But what of the frail 85-year-old who moves slowly but still independently, with a degree of rounded shoulders, small stride, and other mild signs of parkinsonism? Where does normal end and pathologic begin? As a general rule in geriatrics, the distinction between normal and pathologic is based on functional independence. Gait may be the hardest area in which to make that determination.

GAIT EXAMINATION

In clinically assessing gait, one needs to take several things into account. One should look at the tilt of the pelvis, assessing how much the hip moves vertically; the amount of pelvic rotation, or how far the hip moves forward with each stride; the degree of knee flexion; the degree of ankle flexion; and/or the width of the base, or how far apart the feet are placed. These five items are important determinants of the energy consumed in walking.

Arm swing, although not important ergonomically, is very important for diagnosing disorders such as parkinsonism and hemiparesis. Asymmetry or absence of arm swing may point to a developing gait problem even when all other aspects are relatively normal.

Posture is an extremely important and often overlooked aspect of gait. The stooped posture of parkinsonism might appear very similar to that of normal aging, vertebral compression fractures, or ankylosing spondylitis but in context may provide a diagnosis of Parkinson's disease.

Scoliosis (tilting to one side) alters gait as does kyphosis (tilting forward). Either can be the cause of gait dysfunction or itself be the result of a neurologic process causing gait problems. Leaning backward is a rare postural abnormality that may point to dystonia or a psychogenic disorder.

Turning and balance are the final two areas of clinical interest. Does the patient turn en bloc—that is, in one piece (or block)? Balance testing is helpful both for diagnosis as well as for understanding how and why patients fall. In some basal ganglia disorders, balance problems occur early in the disease, before other gait abnormalities are evident, so that the patient walks relatively normally, but balance, if tested, may be impaired. Simple observation does not show this. The patient is first asked to stand with legs together and then after suitable warning, is pulled firmly backward. Normal individuals take one or two steps. Three or four steps is generally abnormal. In some cases the patient would fall if not caught (hence, the examiner must be prepared to catch the patient).

Romberg testing is frequently considered an important sign of balance or cerebellar function by non-neurologists. This test, in which the subject stands with feet together and eyes closed and is observed for sway and loss of balance, was actually intended initially to test posterior spinal cord function for tabes dorsalis (one form of tertiary syphilis). It is now incorrectly interpreted primarily as a cerebellar test. By itself, a positive Romberg—that is, loss of balance—indicates a problem but not what it is. A negative Romberg only eliminates posterior spinal cord dysfunction and none of the common gait and balance disorders. Hence the usefulness of the Romberg test is limited.

Before assessing gait the examiner needs to realize that gait abnormalities may be surprisingly worse than expected from an examination of the seated patient. On one hand, patients with profound hip and thigh weakness may walk surprisingly well once they achieve a standing position, as they mainly need to keep their knees locked to keep from collapsing. They then go forward with calf and foot strength. On the other hand, a patient with a midline cerebellar lesion such as a hemorrhage or tumor may have a normal exam while seated, without evidence of limb ataxia, yet reel like a drunken sailor on standing.

Posture and balance may first be assessed, depending on circumstances, with the patient seated on the examining table, without a back support. Does the patient tend to fall backward or tip to one side? Both are signs of impaired balance and could be evidence of extrapyramidal, cerebellar, or vestibular dysfunction.

Observing the patient stand up is the beginning of the gait assessment. Can the patient stand without using arms to push off? Does standing require more than one attempt? Once the patient is standing, the following aspects should be observed:

1. Posture: Stooped, scoliotic, normal, in extension?
2. Arm swing: Do arms swing? Do they do so equally? Is arm swing excessive or reduced?
3. Base: Normal is shoulder length. Is it too narrow as occurs with spasticity? Is it normal? Is it excessive as occurs with ataxia?
4. Stride length: Is the distance covered normal and is it the same for each foot?
5. Foot strike: Does the heel strike the floor first (normal) or is the strike flat-footed or with the ball of the foot? Do the feet scuff the floor, and if so, is it with the heels, the toes, or one side of the foot?
6. Turn: Does the patient turn normally with a pivot? Is the turn en bloc (in one piece) as in parkinsonism? Is it unsteady?
7. Balance: The patient stands, feet together and eyes open, and after warning, the examiner gives the patient a firm pull from behind. One or two steps is normal. Three or more steps or loss of balance is abnormal.

All of the above are a lot to keep track of. In general, however, we do all of these things unconsciously. Frequently one sees an abnormal gait but cannot determine how it differs from normal. It's just different or odd. Generally, if one breaks walking into its constituent parts, the major different aspects become apparent, pointing to the level of abnormality (i.e., musculoskeletal, peripheral nerve, weakness, ataxia, and so on) or to what areas of the examination need to be performed in a detailed manner.

One can categorize gait abnormalities in a number of ways (Table 5.1). The simplest method is in terms of mechanical disorders and integrative disorders. Mechanical disorders include problems such as arthritis, leg length abnormalities and other deformities, painful joints and limbs, and weakness. Integrative disorders involve an impairment of the normal neurologic process of integrating information from outside the central nervous system and developing and carrying out a plan for walking from point A to point B. Peripheral neuropathies are included in this category because the brain's strategy for dealing with the mismatch of information it receives from the peripheral nerves and the rest of the sensory system (eyes, inner ear, proximal joint position sensors) is not "obvious" to an observer. In contrast, the body's compensation for a foot drop or proximal leg weakness is quite obvious and appears to be a simple mechanical adjustment analogous to the adjustment made for a painful joint.

Gait disorders in the young or middle-aged adult look the same as in the elderly, so they are considered together. Of course the diagnoses have different epidemiologies, but all occur in both groups (e.g., young-onset Parkinson's disease, defined as onset before 40 years of age, afflicts about 5% of people with that disorder). The major difference is that a gray zone exists between the gait change of normal aging, which is associated with a stooped posture, diminished arm swing, diminished stride length, and mild balance problems, and the gait change of Parkinson's disease.

SPECIFIC GAIT DISORDERS

Parkinsonism

Parkinsonism is a generic term meaning "looks like Parkinson's disease." This includes PD and a host of other degenerative processes that

Table 5.1. Neurologic gait disorders

	Posture	Base	Arm Swing	Balance	Description
Parkinsonism	Stooped; flexed at knees, hips, and shoulders	N	↓	↓	Small steps, shuffling
Cerebellar	N	N or ↑	N or ↑	↓	Staggering, "drunk"
Hemiparetic (post–cerebrovascular accident)	N	N	↓ on weak side	N	Weak leg is stiff and circumducts; knee and foot extended
Spastic	N	N or ↓	↑ or ↓	N	Scissoring; knees extended; foot extended; legs circumduct
Foot drop	N	N	N	N	High steps; weak foot hangs
Sensory ataxic	N	.	Abducted	↓	Staggering; "drunk" with slapping steps; much worse with eyes closed
Myopathic	N or hyperlordotic	N	N	N	Waddling; knees locked

N = normal; ↓, decreased; ↑, increased.

all together make up about 20-30% of patients who look like they have PD (excluding patients on drugs that cause parkinsonism). The parkinsonian gait is characterized by a stooped posture, with variable degrees of flexion at all joints. Thus, knees, hips, upper trunk, and neck are all affected. Typically this causes only a round-shouldered posture early on but sometimes one of the other regions will be far more affected. The neck is stiff and hand tremors are frequently accentuated. The stride length is reduced and the heel strike on advancing the feet may be lost, causing shuffling. There is a decrease in arm swing, usually asymmetric. Turning occurs en bloc and generally with several steps rather than a pivot. There is loss of a smooth flow in the overall gestalt, and walking is slower than normal. Balance may be impaired so that the response to being pulled backward is several steps or even loss of balance that would lead to a fall if the patient were not caught. When the patient stands up, he or she may need to use the arms to push off and often fails to put the feet back under the chair. On sitting, the patient may fall like a rock, rather than gently positioning himself or herself in the chair. Distances for sitting are frequently misjudged so that the patient stops too far from the chair or sits down without getting all of the rear-end onto the seat.

Spastic Paraparetic

Cervical myelopathies due to compression of the spinal cord from cervical spondylosis cause gait and usually an associated bladder dysfunction. The bladder dysfunction begins as urinary urgency and frequency but culminates in incontinence as the time from sensing the need to void until the bladder reflexively contracts and empties decreases. In conjunction with this, the compression of the corticospinal tracts in the neck causes spasticity in the legs, initially without weakness. The gait dysfunction is due to the spasticity. The knees and ankles become increasingly stiff in extension. Thus, the knee tends to lose its flexion and the foot starts to extend when brought forward instead of flexing. First the heel strike is lost, then the foot strikes with the ball of the foot. Shoes wear out in the front. Along with the increased tone causing extension of the knee and ankle, the abductors of the thighs become tighter, causing excessive narrowing at the base. The legs tend to scissor. Arm swing may remain normal or even increase, to attempt to "pull" the legs forward to compensate for the reduced stride, the scraping of the feet, and the slowing. One further observation concerns leg movement. Since the leg is stiff in extension and the abductors are pulling, the leg moves in a curvilinear fashion. It cannot simply be moved forward as the floor is in the way. The leg goes forward and out, and once it passes the plane of the other leg, it goes inward toward the midline. The ability to recover from lost balance is reduced because the legs are slow and clumsy, reflecting the spasticity.

The diagnosis is made clinically with the demonstration of spastic legs, with an increase in leg tone when the knees are quickly but passively moved (see Appendix 1 on the neurologic exam), increased deep tendon reflexes, and usually positive Babinski reflexes. The patient is slow, with toe tapping, and somewhat clumsy. The neurologic exam from the waist up is normal. The laboratory study of choice is magnetic resonance imaging of the cervical cord. However, clinically one cannot usually distinguish a cervical and thoracic cord problem unless sensory signs or symptoms are present to localize the level.

Hemiparetic

The hemiparetic gait syndrome is the typical post-stroke gait. The most obvious characteristic is the asymmetry. One arm swings and the other does not. One leg moves normally while the other is spastic. The stride lengths are different.

After a typical stroke causing weakness, there is an increase in tone on the affected side. This tone increase parallels the distribution of the weakness itself. In most cases the "antigravity" muscles, which are extensors, are weakened more than the flexors (triceps more affected than biceps, wrist extensors more affected than flexors, grip more affected than finger extensors). As the tone increases over the next few weeks, the arm becomes increasingly flexed, at the elbow, wrist, and grip, as well as being adducted (held close to the chest) at the shoulder. The leg, in contrast, as with the spastic gait described above, becomes stiff in extension. This is obviously a useful adaptive development since the leg acts as its own cane. The knee is stiff in extension, allowing the leg to support the weight but causing circumduction.

Ataxic Gait

Ataxia is a term that has defied accurate description. An ataxic gait is clumsy and irregular, with a degree of randomness that reflects balance as the primary problem. There are three major causes of ataxic gait: cerebellar dysfunction, vestibular dysfunction, and sensory neuropathy. Clinically only the sensory ataxic gait can be reliably distinguished from the other two, while cerebellar and vestibular gait disorders look identical since their fundamental problem is the same.

Although medical students are generally taught that cerebellar gait disorders produce a wide base, this is not always true. The base may be wide or normal (never too narrow), but with walking there will be staggering and a tendency either to veer to one side or to meander from one side to the other. An inebriated person usually walks this way. The person has a normal base but has a forward propulsion, then moves first to one side, then to the other, with an unsteady momentum and a variable risk of falling due to imbalance. Unilateral cerebellar lesions will usually cause staggering to the side of the lesion.

Vestibular dysfunction is associated with vertigo if only one labyrinth is affected. When both are affected, however, there is no vertigo. The patient's sense of balance is impaired proportionately to the extent of the labyrinthine dysfunction. As with midline cerebellar lesions, tests of leg strength and agility are normal. The base may be wide and the patient staggers to one side, if one labyrinth is affected, or to either side if both are.

Sensory ataxia looks different from the other two ataxic gait syndromes only because there is usually a high-stepping, foot-slapping quality added to the ataxic qualities. The central nervous system, seemingly because it is not fully aware of where the feet and the ground are, adjusts to step over imaginary objects and then to slap the floor as if to strengthen the sensory input telling it where the floor is. The result from the Romberg test should be positive.

Examining any ataxic gait requires a good sensory evaluation of the feet, in particular to assess distal sensation for touch and pinprick and, more important, to position sense. Disorders such as tabes dorsalis and subacute combined degeneration (vitamin B_{12} deficiency) produce position sense loss due to the degeneration of the posterior columns of the spinal cord and while rare today, are treatable.

Antalgic Gait

Antalgic gait refers to gait abnormalities due to pain. Active arthritis in the hips, knees, and ankles or painful disorders of the feet leads to a variety of different adaptations in the attempt to reduce pain. Patients may limp, transfer weight from one side to the other in a rapid manner, or simply alter their posture to seek some means of pain reduction. In all cases, this information is ascertained by questioning the patient.

Multifactorial Gait Abnormality

Multifactorial gait abnormality describes the broad spectrum of gait disorders seen in many elderly patients. These patients often suffer a variety of relatively minor disorders that have an impact on gait. The hypertensive, arthritic, diabetic, obese patient with cataracts, for example, has a sensory neuropathy of mild proportions, with joint pain, impaired vision, excess spine strain from obesity, and possibly old stroke. Each item by itself might not cause any problem but, when added to the others, becomes synergistic as the various compensating mechanisms are each affected. These patients tend to have parkinsonian features but clearly do not have Parkinson's disease. They may be a bit stooped, have reduced balance and arm swing, and take small steps.

Senile Gait

Senile gait has become a less acceptable term over the past decade. Certainly many observational data indicate that aging alone—that is, in the absence of pathology—produces mild parkinsonian changes. Aging is also associated, however, with mild peripheral sensory changes, decline in vestibular function, and diminished muscle mass, strength, and speed. Whether a change is pathologic or not may be impossible to determine until time has passed and the process of normal aging separates from the expected course of a pathologic process.

Fear of Falling

One fall, or even just the fear of falling, may induce a pathologic gait. Such patients often walk as if on ice, with excessive slowness, placing each foot flat on the ground before advancing the next. In many cases some degree of fear is reasonable, but the fear itself actually worsens the gait and balance in a manner quite similar to the difficulty a person with fear of heights might experience on a mountain rock climb. The treatment is aggressive but supportive physical therapy once a complete evaluation finds no other explanation.

Normal Pressure Hydrocephalus

Normal pressure hydrocephalus is a rare but often-discussed problem causing a gait disorder that has been described in so many contradictory terms that one must conclude that the spectrum of gaits is very broad. Mostly it is considered a form of "parkinsonism from the waist down" (i.e., with small shuffling steps, turning en bloc, and poor balance, but normal base, normal or increased arm swing, and normal posture). Ataxic gait and freezing, however, have also been described.

Factitious Gait Disorder

Factitious gait disorder is a broad range of phenomenology that should be considered when the history and examination do not make sense. The diagnosis should always be confirmed by a gait specialist because some rare neurologic disorders, especially dystonia and episodic non-seizure movement disorders accepted as "organic," are frequently misdiagnosed as psychogenic.

The observation of *la belle indifférence* and hysterical personality is not present in most cases. There may or may not be a clear psychiatric history or psychological precipitant. The standard teaching that psychogenic disorders do not cause injuries is false, so the presence of a fracture or a broken tooth does not militate against diagnosis but does reinforce the need for an expert opinion.

Generally these disorders appear suddenly, often exacerbate and remit (unlike most disorders that are slowly progressive), and have an unusual appearance. They occur at younger ages than most gait disorders and may produce disability shortly after onset. Neurologic evaluation is generally much more helpful than a psychiatric examination as the latter needs the former to diagnose and then treat this conversion disorder.

CLINICAL PEARLS

- Falls, as distinguished from trips and faints, should always be considered symptoms of significant pathology and require evaluation.
- Any gait abnormality must have a documented explanation. If a patient requires a cane or walker, the reason should be recorded, whether it is arthritis, hip fracture, or bunions. If the gait abnormality cannot be adequately explained (i.e., there is no pain, obvious leg length inequality, or scoliosis), then a neurologist should evaluate the patient.

6

Memory Loss,
Cognitive Dysfunction,
and Mental Status Changes

Mental status abnormalities may be considered in a number of ways.
For clinical purposes, the most important ways are the nature of the
change and the time course. Mental changes can be crudely divided
into behavioral changes, cognitive changes, and memory changes.
Behavioral changes affect personality and mood and include depression, irritability, lability, mania, and sexual alterations. Cognitive decline
means loss of integrative and problem-solving skills, or loss of intelligence in general. Memory dysfunction cannot occur in isolation. Poor
memory impedes intellectual function, yet there are patients whose
memory is so much worse than their overall intellectual function that
we can consider it almost as a separate function, as in Korsakoff's psychosis. The mental changes that occur most frequently are the dementias. These develop over periods of months to years and only rarely
over periods measured in weeks. Behavioral changes may be part of
dementing processes, primary psychiatric problems, or secondary to
nondementing organic disorders and may develop over days to years.
Memory problems, with rare exceptions, develop over months.

HISTORY

The history of behavioral change often puts the disorder into its
proper medical context. An abrupt change occurring over seconds or
minutes suggests an acute brain disorder such as a stroke or seizure.

Something developing over hours to days suggests a subacute
process, usually an organic encephalopathy such as viral encephalitis,
drug effect, neuroendocrine disturbance, liver or renal failure, or
electrolyte imbalance. A slowly progressive disorder developing over
months points to a slow brain process such as a degenerative condition or tumor.

Primary psychiatric conditions vary in terms of how quickly
they develop and, like medical disorders, have distinct ages of
onset. For example, patients who develop schizophrenia are almost
young adults or teenagers. Newly developed psychotic behavior in
a 60- or 70-year-old is never due to schizophrenia. Depression may
occur at any age and is slow in development, occurring over days
to months. Mania may develop quickly but usually occurs in someone with a history of depression and is not likely to present in an
elderly person.

The history of someone with a mental status derangement often
has to be pieced together. The patient is frequently unable to supply
reliable information. The family often fails to notice odd behavior,
either thinking it normal or a personal idiosyncrasy. Thus, a family
describes a sudden change when an elderly parent leaves the house
naked, whereas they had failed to be concerned when she had been
unable to consistently find her room or dress herself for months.
Careful history taking is crucial. Did manic-type behavior develop
suddenly or was it related to the psychiatric admission for a nervous
breakdown 10 years before? Family history is very important in
diagnosing affective disorders. Determining the patient's level of
function in very concrete terms (did he read the newspaper, drive a
car, buy his own food, or cook on his own?) is often crucial. A problem I often run into and discuss in more detail later is differentiating
between Alzheimer's disease (AD) and a Wernicke's type (fluent)
aphasia. Although a skilled examiner may be able to do this, I cannot
always. Thus, I rely heavily on the history (a computed tomography
[CT] scan of the brain may not reveal the small but devastating Wernicke's area stroke).

DEMENTIA

Dementia is a general term that describes a decline in intellectual function from baseline. *Dementia* was called *senility* in the past, but as increasing numbers of people have reached old age, and as people's sensitivity to language has increased, the term *senile* is now outdated (along with words like *idiot*). The term *dementia* does not imply a particular cause and is to be distinguished from delirium, a condition characterized by impaired attention and inability to maintain a train of thought due to thought intrusions or hallucinations. In dementia, the variability of mental state from hour to hour is less than with delirium, and although the patient is distractible, the patient's thought process is clear until distraction arises. In delirium the distractions are self-generated whereas the demented have a reasonable ability to focus if examined in a quiet setting.

There are numerous causes for dementia, most of which occur in old age. AD is certainly the number one cause of dementia in the Western world, with vascular dementia and the Lewy body variant of AD causing most of the remaining cases of dementia. AD affects about 10% of Americans older than 65, making it about 10 times as common as Parkinson's disease (PD). It afflicts about 45% of people older than age 85. One small report in 1998 noted that every person above age 100 in a Dutch city was demented, although not all had AD. In the United States about 55–70% of dementia is ascribed to AD.

While treatment is still in its infancy, the accuracy of diagnosis of dementing illness is unimportant as long as the illness is accurately categorized as a reversible or irreversible disorder. In the future, when disease-specific therapy is available, accurate diagnosis will be required.

Alzheimer's Disease

AD is the most important dementing illness and, like other neurodegenerative disorders, is undoubtedly a mixture of related diseases that cause similar clinical and pathologic disorders. Whereas the cause of most cases of AD is unknown, at least three distinct genes on different chromosomes have been found in families with inherited forms of AD. The pathologies are similar and there are common features of these diseases, making the single term *AD* acceptable even though their genetic bases are different. Whether most or even all forms of AD are inherited is difficult to determine because the onset is so late that parents of probands are usually dead and may have died before the disease could be manifest.

AD usually begins as a memory disorder, with recent memory affected before the older ones. Family members will say of a patient that he is "sharp as a tack, he remembers things from 50 years ago like it was yesterday," but he gets lost a lot, misplaces things, and keeps asking the same questions repeatedly. Early on the patient has some insight into the problem and may keep lists or limit activities to avoid embarrassment. Whereas a variety of behavioral changes occur with later stages, depression is a common early feature and often leads to the clinical question (discussed later) of whether the patient is pseudodemented due to depression, which is reversible, or depressed in association with dementia. Usually both are present, but treatment of the former improves the latter. Over time other changes develop along with the increasing memory problems. In neurobehavioral parlance, dementias are often divided into the two major categories of cortical and subcortical variants. AD is the paradigmatic cortical dementia. Both types involve progressive amnesia. The cortical dementias cause loss of cognitive functions that are usually impaired only with direct damage to the cortex, such as aphasia and apraxia. One major hallmark of AD is impaired language function. Formal language testing, even in the office setting, usually brings out problems of word finding (e.g., point to 10 objects, such as ear, nose, eyebrow, lip, chin, two or three fingers, knuckles, lapel, and shoelace), comprehension for three-step commands or complex sentences ("Put the comb next to the tissue and then put the cup on the tissue"), or writing. Having the patient write two or three educationally appropriate sentences tests the patient and also provides a benchmark for future comparisons. Constructional apraxia, with impaired clock drawing, poor figure copying, and so on, also provides written benchmarks for future comparisons as well as current assessments. These types of problems are usually not apparent to the family because most daily interactions are social and highly routine activities that require few modifications. Often, because social graces are well preserved, the family fails to realize how little is actually understood when they use complex ideas or complex sentences.

With lost insight comes impaired judgment that leads to a set of behavioral problems. The patient who denies a memory problem cannot understand why the car keys are not where they were left. He or she cannot recall getting lost. Those patients are often dangerous because they leave things cooking on the range, water running in the sink, doors and windows open, and so forth. Behavioral issues may emerge with major personality transformations. With depression or memory impairment comes irritability and lability. Loss of inhibition may range from mildly inappropriate statements ("How are you feeling today?" may get the response, "I'd be okay if it wasn't for you") to grossly abnormal behaviors like undressing in front of company. Paranoia is a common accompaniment to memory loss; objects misplaced are presumed stolen, workers in the house are burglars, and so forth. Noises in the house from the caregiver are perceived to be caused by thieves so the patient calls the police. Family members are believed to be impostors, which prevents caregiving until the patient can be redirected. With enough time, patients lose their emotions and become abulic, or lacking in emotions. They become increasingly withdrawn. Distinguishing this from depression is not easy, and it should be treated as depression if the diagnosis is unsure, because depression is treatable and abulia is not. Demented, abulic patients look like the characters in the movie *Invasion of the Body Snatchers*. The one comforting thought is that the patient is no longer suffering because he or she has lost all mental capacity.

AD does not cause focal neurologic signs. These, if present, have another explanation or the patient does not have AD. Having one neurologic disease does not preclude a second. People with strokes or PD also develop AD and vice versa. However, it is common for the more advanced AD patient to develop features of PD, without tremor, even without any exposure to antipsychotic drugs. AD is associated with an increased frequency of seizures and also myoclonus. The latter occasionally causes some concern over a possible diagnosis of Creutzfeldt-Jacob disease but is usually a late element in the disease, occurring several years into the course.

The diagnosis of AD is still a clinical one and is based primarily on exclusionary criteria. The current criteria for the diagnosis of probable AD includes a documented decline in two or more areas of cognition, an abnormal score on some generally accepted dementia scale, progressive memory loss, onset between ages 40 and 90, normal level of alertness, and absence of other disorders that could explain the syndrome. Supportive data for the diagnosis include a positive family history, language or praxis deficits, problems with behavior or activities of daily life, and normal routine laboratory studies. Laboratory studies that are recommended to exclude potentially reversible conditions include a brain imaging study, generally a computed tomography (CT) scan but possibly magnetic resonance imaging (MRI); measurement of vitamin B_{12} levels; Venereal Disease Research Laboratory testing; measurement of folate levels; routine blood chemistry profile; thyroid function tests; and complete blood count. Brain imaging shows atrophy that is often appropriate for age but may also reveal unsuspected pathology that may or may not be coincidental. Electroencephalography is not useful and either shows no abnormality or diffuse slowing. Spinal fluid is normal and is not obtained except in exceptional circumstances. Brain single-photon emission computed tomography scanning may show decreased perfusion in the temporoparietal regions, a nonspecific but supportive finding. Laboratory tests currently being marketed to diagnose AD are not yet generally accepted. None can be used to make a definite diagnosis; all are considered supportive diagnostic criteria.

Management is predominantly symptom oriented. Two drugs that block the breakdown of acetylcholine, tacrine and donepezil, mildly improve memory by acting as cholinergic-enhancing agents. Both work only to a mild degree and only in some patients. Tacrine is associated with a high percentage of liver toxicity whereas donepezil is quite benign. The challenge of management, however, is the control of behavioral problems and counseling the family on current and future problems. The behavioral issues are depression, disinhibition, and psychosis. Altered sleep habits are extremely disruptive for family caregivers. Depression is treated with low doses of antidepressants. The newer class of serotonin reuptake inhibitors such as fluoxetine, sertraline, and paroxetine is well tolerated and does not generally trigger mental side effects. Typical antipsychotics such as haloperidol are widely used but frequently induce parkinsonism, which leads to falls and immobility, or occasionally induce akathisia, an intolerable restlessness that exacerbates all the behavioral problems. I recommend low doses of an atypical antipsychotic such as quetiapine, olanzapine, or clozapine if an antipsychotic is required. The fact that a drug is used to treat psychosis does not mean that it cannot itself worsen the confusion. Most of the antipsychotics, especially the new atypical drugs, have multiple neurotransmitter effects, sometimes including anticholinergic ones that can worsen memory or attention or cause sedation-induced cognitive declines. Thus, the antipsychotic itself may cause delirium, which is one reason that all psychoactive drugs must be initiated at low doses.

The sleep problem is usually one of the most difficult to solve. Patients may go to sleep appropriately but awaken in the middle of the night and wander, perhaps getting dressed and going outside or doing something equally inappropriate. Trazodone, a sedating antidepressant, is one drug to consider if a sedating antipsychotic is not already in use. The benzodiazepines may also be used, and obviously the trade-off in terms of worsened cognitive function and balance must be weighed against the sleep benefit for the patient and family. Whether melatonin will play a role here is not yet known.

Dementia with Lewy Bodies

The term *dementia with Lewy bodies* is an addition to the medical lexicon officially originating in 1995. Before that time, the more generic terms of *diffuse Lewy body disease* and the *Lewy body vari-*

ant of Alzheimer's disease were used. The explosion of interest in this little-known entity is quite instructive because it teaches us to be cautious in our reliance even on our histopathologic interpretations of neurodegenerative diseases.

Lewy bodies are eosinophilic cytoplasmic inclusions found in the degenerating pigmented brain stem cells in PD. These are mainly found in the substantia nigra but are in other brain stem locations in PD as well. In 1960, in a routine autopsy, Lewy bodies were identified for the first time in the cortex as well. Until the mid-1980s, the occurrence of Lewy bodies in the cortex was considered rare and material for isolated case reports. The entity was labeled *diffuse Lewy body disease*. Then an autopsy study from England concluded that diffuse Lewy body disease was the second most common cause of dementia in an English district. With the special stain ubiquitin, many Lewy bodies could be identified that were not seen with routine hematoxylin and eosin staining. Thus, with a minor improvement in staining and greater attention to this part of the brain, a relatively newly recognized entity, considered extremely rare, turned out to be the second most common etiology for dementia in the Western world. This type of observation certainly undermines our security about any classification system not based on genetic or biochemical criteria. (This, incidentally, brings to mind recent improvements in staining that demonstrate that virtually all neurodegenerative disorders contain cytoplasmic inclusions, a fact that has emerged only in the last few years.)

Dementia with Lewy bodies is thought to account for 15–25% of all dementias in Western countries. Thus, it stands behind AD and ahead of vascular dementia in prevalence. Its existence both complicates and eases our clinical decision making. By providing a new diagnostic category that is actually common, it allows diagnoses of more patients than before. On the other hand, the amount of overlap between this entity, PD with dementia, AD, and AD with parkinsonian features undermines much of our diagnostic confidence. At this time, with no cure, no ability to slow progression, and meager symptomatic treatment, the problem is more academic than real, but in the future there will be treatment options and having a correct diagnosis will most likely be a major determinant in the treatment response. That is, there will likely be different treatments for the dementia of AD and Lewy body disease; not all patients will simply be placed on cholinesterase inhibitors.

Lewy body disease causes a variable type of dementia with or without cortical features such as aphasia or apraxia, but that typically causes memory and executive dysfunction typical of subcortical dementias. Memory traces are usually present but cues need to be given, unlike AD, in which the memory slate remains blank and priming does not help. Cognition slows down so that there may be a few seconds required to answer questions. Concentration and sequencing tasks are both disturbed. However, the major distinctions between Lewy body disease and AD are the presence of visual hallucinations unrelated to the use of drugs that affect over 60% of patients with Lewy body disease. Delusions, sometimes paranoid in nature, are common, again unrelated to medications. The onset of the dementia is typically more rapid than in AD and fluctuations in attention and level of arousal are common. Some patients have periods of confusion lasting minutes to hours alternating with periods of lucidity. Daytime sleepiness is also common. Patients with Lewy body disease are thought to be at more risk of autonomic dysfunction than are patients with other dementing illnesses, making them presumably more likely to suffer syncopal spells. Because there are also Lewy bodies in the substantia nigra associated with cortical degenerating neurons, parkinsonism also is seen but may appear late.

In brief, Lewy body disease patients may have what looks like typical PD but have an early onset of dementia characterized by fluctuating degrees of confusion, alertness, or psychosis, with visual hallucinations not due to anti-PD medications. Other types of hallucinations may also occur.

The main differential diagnostic list is AD and PD. Many AD patients develop parkinsonism, but it occurs late in the course, when dementia is severe. The AD dementia is slower in progression. AD fluctuations are typically of the sun-downing type, with consistently worsening behavior in the evening. Hallucinations are less common than delusions and the dementia typically involves language function and praxis. PD is associated with dementia in about 20–30% of cases, and the pathologic substrate is not well understood. This dementia is always a late feature that occurs years after the parkinsonism and is seen generally once the motor signs become prominent. It may be difficult to clinically distinguish Lewy body disease from the combined effect of PD with AD.

The parkinsonism of LBD appears to respond to the same medications that are used in PD, but the anti-PD medications are more likely to induce visual hallucinations and psychosis than is PD.

Treatment for the dementia is unknown. Although one may try the cholinesterase inhibitors, which increase acetylcholine function, this theoretically could (and in limited clinical experience does) worsen parkinsonism. Drugs that block acetylcholine are used to treat the symptoms of PD and are helpful especially in relieving tremors, so that drugs that do the opposite may cause opposite effects. Data on the efficacy and side effects of these drugs in LBD are minimal. Certainly they are worth considering, but attention must focus on functional benefit versus side effects. Vitamin E and selegiline have no proved value in this syndrome. In both PD and AD their benefit, if any, is small, but vitamin E is inexpensive and free of side effects. Selegiline may cause side effects, especially orthostatic hypotension and worsened behavior. In AD these drugs were shown to delay time until nursing home placement but not dementia progression.

Vascular Dementia

Vascular dementia is a nonspecific term that describes at least two types of pathologic entities leading to dementia. One is a time-honored, well-understood process: multi-infarct dementia (MID). The other is not understood and is in transition, occurring primarily as an MRI diagnosis.

MID describes a dementing illness due to multiple strokes. With each stroke the patient suddenly either develops new focal abnormalities, as is typical with strokes, or undergoes a sudden worsening of the dementia even in the absence of new focal signs. There is then a several days' or a few weeks' recovery period, as is true after strokes in general. Thus, the clinical picture is one of a step-like decline followed by stable or mildly improved function until the next sudden decline. Patients usually have focal abnormalities on examination due to strokes affecting motor function in some way, from mild clumsiness or weakness on one side to reflex asymmetries and positive Babinski reflexes. These findings correlate with the loci of the strokes. Multiple lacunar infarcts, usually occurring deep in the brain, cause a pseudobulbar palsy (*pseudobulbar* means it simulates weakness in bulbar, or medulla, functions, which are swallowing, gag reflex, and tongue movements) with an associated behavior abnormality: labile emotions, slurred speech, and swallowing problems. The emotional lability of these patients is an interesting phenomenon because the patients are often aware of it. They may complain that they laugh or cry for little or even no apparent reason and find it very disturbing. It is involuntary, and the patient's inner emotional state is often not congruent with the apparent affect. However, while interesting, this problem is not diagnostic of MID and may occur without dementia or with other dementias, but its presence should make the diagnosis of MID a consideration.

A CT scan should reveal infarcts but often reveals diffuse atrophy, possibly asymmetric, depending on the distribution of strokes. MRI is by far the better diagnostic study because it is much less likely to miss small strokes. One frequently sees a CT showing large ventricles and large sulci but no strokes, while the MRI shows a myriad of small infarcts as the cause of the diffuse atrophy.

There is no treatment for this type of dementia. Reducing stroke risk is clearly the only intervention currently available, and this presumably only slows disease progression rather than reversing any symptoms.

Non-MID Vascular Dementia

Non-MID vascular dementia is relatively new terrain, brought to light by MRI. The brain MRI is a very sensitive test that all too often produces small, patchy white-matter lesions initially called unidentified bright objects, seen on the T_2-enhanced images. At autopsy the pathology reveals patchy demyelination, gliosis, and shrunken vessels surrounded by cerebrospinal fluid, all of which T_2 enhance. This process is thought to occur on the basis of ischemia, but this hypothesis is unproved. There is a clear association between these T_2 patches and hypertension and diabetes, as well as stroke, supporting the ischemia concept. The notion of slowly progressive ischemic deficits evolving over weeks, months, or years that this concept implies, however, runs counter to all previous neurologic teaching that strokes are sudden events and that insufficient blood flow produces a sudden deficit or a faint, not a slowly progressive, disorder. These patchy areas are in the white matter, and, when large, are inseparable radiographically from stroke. MRI reports generally describe these as areas of demyelination consistent with microvascular disease, ischemic changes, or multiple sclerosis. The lesions may occur as tiny volumes, larger patches, or confluent regions around the lateral ventricles. Around the ventricles, the increased T_2 signal is more likely due to extravasated cerebrospinal fluid (CSF) than demyelination. Presumably, small arterioles shrivel up due to hypertension or diabetes, and CSF exits the ventricle to produce microscopic puddles of CSF that light up on MRI.

Much research focuses on these T_2-enhancing patches. Their occurrence correlates with dementia, depression, gait dysfunction, and other central nervous system dysfunction as well, suggesting that the MRI lesions are not benign even if they do not represent strokes. Many neurologists believe that these lesions interfere with normal brain function and that their volume and distribution determine the clinical problems. Thus, lesions in one set of locations cause dementia or gait dysfunction.

Non-MID vascular dementia is sometimes distinguished from a rare disorder called *Binswanger's disease* in which frank strokes occurring at the gray matter–white matter junction produce a clinical picture of dementia and gait dysfunction.

WERNICKE'S APHASIA

Wernicke's aphasia is the paradigmatic fluent aphasia. It usually occurs as the result of a very small but devastating stroke and is a frequent cause of acute confusional state in the elderly because it is often not accompanied by weakness other than mild facial weakness. Occasionally, such patients are misdiagnosed as being psychotic or demented. They have severely impaired comprehension and produce a babbling type of speech that at first sounds normal but with closer attention is empty and meaningless. It often contains neologisms, or new words, that sound like real words but are not. Their grammar seems normal and articulation is also normal. If the fluent aphasia occurs in a language unknown to the examiner, it sounds like normal speech. The family of the patient, however, can report that the speech makes no sense. Patients have no insight into their problem and behave as if they understand what was said and were understood in turn. Initially their affect is surprisingly happy and unconcerned. The more impaired they are, the happier they seem. Some patients become extremely verbal and talk incessantly. Aside from this extraordinary language problem and the associated lack of insight, behavior is otherwise unaffected. Patients eat normally, bathe themselves, use the toilet facilities appropriately, and, if hospitalized, do not wander the wards or use fellow patients' belongings. The language disorder is therefore isolated and the usual behavioral and memory problems that one sees with AD do not occur.

In the chronic cases of fluent aphasia—the patient who had the stroke years before and is now being evaluated for the first time— paranoia is common and some recognition of the communication disorder exists. The history is important. Since the onset of the language problem, there should have been no further decline in cognitive or memory function.

Virtually all other aphasias are associated with right-sided weakness and language impairments that are closely identified as organic in etiology.

OTHER MENTAL STATUS ABNORMALITIES

Toxic Mental Status Abnormalities

Reversible causes of mental status changes must always be considered. Routine blood studies exclude electrolyte imbalances such as sodium and calcium problems, renal failure, and glucose abnormalities. Liver failure, delayed drug effects, drug withdrawal, and remote or toxic effects of systemic disease are frequently overlooked for a variety of reasons. A mental status change without a new focal neurologic sign should always point to this broad classification.

Hepatic encephalopathy usually occurs in the setting of a patient with known liver disease or in a patient with clear evidence of liver failure, with elevated liver enzymes, hyperbilirubinemia with jaundice, and possibly elevated serum ammonia. However, this is not always the case. When the liver becomes mostly cirrhotic, liver enzymes and bilirubin may be normal. Ammonia may or may not be elevated. Patients may have an elevated prothrombin time due to failure of the liver to produce clotting factors. In addition, there is usually a respiratory alkalosis induced by hyperventilation (in the absence of a pulmonary disease such as pneumonia). Patients are usually apathetic, lethargic, and confused. Asterixis, when present, is a useful sign. It is elicited by having the patient sustain a muscle contraction for several seconds. Usually the hands and feet are extended and a typical flap occurs due to brief relaxation of the contracting muscle. Although many students learn to "test" for asterixis on comatose patients, it cannot be done. The patient must be contracting muscles voluntarily. Sometimes the proximal arms are affected, producing large, jerky movements. Brain MRI frequently reveals a T_1 signal in the basal ganglia and brain stem (in contrast to almost all other processes that produce T_2 signals).

Drug-induced mental side effects usually occur soon after the offending drug is started, but not always. For example, L-dopa used in PD may be tolerated for years before causing hallucinations or psychosis. Thus, older patients, particularly those who have been taking stable doses of anxiolytics or antidepressants, may develop mental changes due to possibly diminished brain flexibility. Many physicians assume that if a drug regimen is stable and has been tolerated for months or years, then it could not be the problem. This is incorrect.

Possibly the most common cause of acute or subacute mental decline in the elderly is a systemic illness, particularly an infection. I have seen patients admitted for evaluation of stupor eventually ascribed to cholecystitis, pneumonia, or urinary tract infection. Other inflammatory illnesses such as collagen vascular disorders can do the same, as can systemic viral syndromes.

Pathologists in recent years have claimed that autopsies reveal a surprisingly high percentage of cases with evidence of the Wernicke-Korsakoff syndrome, but this may be exaggerated. It should be considered, however, in all patients with unexplained stupor and a global confusional state. Although medical students are taught to look for severe recent memory loss and confabulation, these are not usually present early on, or at least not out of proportion to the degree of confusion. Obviously these patients do not have measurable alcohol levels so that the syndrome is diagnosed on clinical grounds alone. Thus, thiamine should be given to these patients.

Any patient with new-onset confusion, especially if stuporous and without focal neurological signs, requires metabolic studies including electrolytes, glucose, calcium, renal and liver function tests, complete blood count with differential, prothrombin time, thyroid-stimulating hormone, chest x-ray, urinalysis, and erythrocyte sedimentation rate tests. If the neck is stiff on flexion or the patient is febrile without a clear source, a lumbar puncture is required.

PSYCHIATRIC ILLNESSES

Psychiatric illnesses are always a consideration in explaining mental status changes. Depression is the most common and is recognized by a sad affect, lack of self-worth, guilt feelings, decreased energy, decreased appetite with weight loss, and decreased sleeping at night. These are frequently associated with multiple somatic symptoms. One of the most common symptoms is memory loss or frank dementia. When this intellectual impairment is due completely to the depression, it is termed *pseudodementia* because it is fully reversible. In actual practice some degree of pseudodementia is common, but in most cases there is an underlying true organic dementia that is exacerbated by the depression.

It is very common for patients with early or moderate dementia to also be depressed, creating the question of dementia, pseudodementia, or both. The most appropriate approach is to treat the depression and see what happens.

The sudden onset of a major behavioral change is uncommon in primary psychiatric disorders. Psychotic disorders typically evolve over days to weeks and even then are preceded by behaviors that are clearly unusual, although not so much as to draw too much attention. Mania may arise suddenly, and a first episode, by definition, seemingly occurs out of the blue, but a sudden onset is uncommon.

Like neurologic disorders, psychiatric diagnoses occur at certain ages. Schizophrenia is a disease that begins in young adulthood. Childhood-onset or late adult-onset schizophrenia are both very rare. Most schizophrenics have become psychotic as young adults, most commonly in their late teens or early 20s. Depression may develop at any age but only rarely has psychotic features. Manic depression is an uncommon disorder that virtually never presents in old age. Generally it develops in young and middle-aged adults. Onset of mania may be relatively abrupt, developing over days, and may be difficult for nonpsychiatrists to distinguish from a schizophrenic with an agitated psychosis.

CLINICAL PEARLS

- Prolonged amnestic spells lasting hours, during which the subject carries on in an apparently normal fashion but is then amnestic, are always due to a psychogenic origin or to occult intoxication.
- Patients who complain of memory dysfunction probably do not have such a condition. Usually depression or anxiety is the explanation for this problem that often represents diminished attention.
- Prolonged (hours-long) spells of altered behavior may be due to occult intoxications even when the patient comes for diagnosis.
- Auditory hallucinations are generally due to primary psychiatric problems (except alcohol hallucinosis), whereas visual hallucinations are usually of toxic origin (narcotics, L-dopa, and so on).
- Delirium tremens usually begin about 3 days after the last alcoholic drink.
- Weight gain as a symptom of depression occurs most frequently in young women. Other groups who are depressed lose weight.

7

Disorders of Vision and Other Special Senses

VISUAL DISORDERS

Most visual problems are not neurologic in origin. Distinguishing neurologic from ophthalmologic problems accelerates treatment greatly because emergency outpatient consultations are often difficult to obtain and thus cause delays. Reviewing a few basic principles helps localize the cause of a vision problem and gets the patient to the correct consultant expeditiously.

The eye perceives light through the retina, which then transmits data back to the brain via the optic nerve. One optic nerve transmits all the information from one eye. The two optic nerves merge to form the optic chiasm. Lesions of one optic nerve thus cause monocular visual problems. At the chiasm, each optic nerve splits into two equal parts so that the optic tract on the brain side of the chiasm contains information concerning the contralateral visual field from each eye. Immediately on entering the brain, the optic tract synapses and sends the optic radiation to the occipital cortex.

Vascular disease affects vision by affecting either the eye, the optic nerve, the optic radiations, or the visual (occipital) cortex. Loss of vision in one eye implies a problem in the optic nerve or the eye. Visual loss in the same visual field in each eye indicates a problem in the brain. A lesion in the optic chiasm, where the optic nerves cross, produces a temporal field cut on both sides.

Blurred vision is usually due to a refraction problem. Only two neurologic problems cause blurred vision: inflammation of the optic nerve and dysconjugate eye movements. A host of eye disorders that are generally slowly progressive, such as cataracts and glaucoma (which rarely can be acute), cause blurred vision as well. Inflammatory disorders of the eye develop more rapidly but are less common. They are not sudden in onset like vascular disorders.

Blurred Vision

Extraocular Muscle Weakness

Blurred vision caused by extraocular muscle weakness is actually misperceived diplopia. When two images are seen very closely together, the image is blurred. When the two images are far apart, two distinct images are seen. This is very clear on television sets, when ghost images appear. When the ghost is close to the real image, only one blurred image is perceived. Usually the history solves this problem because this type of blurred vision resolves when either eye is closed, removing one of the images. Patients often keep one eye closed to maintain acuity at the expense of visual field. The patient is not able to determine which eye is the weak one because each image looks normal. The most peripheral image (farthest from center) arises from the weaker eye.

Brain problems do not cause blurred vision other than through extraocular muscle weakness. Thus, if blurring does not improve on closing one eye, the problem is either in the optic nerve or the eye itself. In these cases, one eye perceives blurred images and the other eye is normal.

Optic Nerve Dysfunction

Unlike a refractive error, in which light is distorted on entering the eye, an optic nerve lesion produces alterations of the electrical impulses from the retina. This results in reduced acuity and reduced brightness of color vision. This disruption may be partial or complete and cannot be corrected. An analogy between the visual problems caused by the lens (refractive error) versus the optic nerve might be the difference between the image produced by a poor-quality printer that smudges and a circuit problem in the computer itself. Thus, if the blurred vision is correctable with lenses or use of a pinhole, then the problem is refractive.

Optic nerve lesions are highly variable in location, size, and severity. A severe lesion of one section of the nerve produces blindness, whereas a small disruption in one restricted region causes only mildly impaired visual input to the brain. If severe enough, an afferent pupillary defect is evident. This is also called a *Marcus-Gunn pupil* and is demonstrated by what is termed the *swinging flashlight test*. A bright light is pointed at one eye. If it is the good eye, the brain receives a 100% stimulus. If it is the affected eye, only a fraction, say 50%, of the light impulse reaches the brain because the affected optic nerve does not convey all the retinal impulses. Because the pupil size is determined by the brain, which integrates information from both sides, both pupils always remain an equal size. Thus, if the bad eye receives the light first, then both pupils constrict. Then the light swings to the good eye, which perceives the same light as being brighter, and causes both pupils to contract more. When the flashlight then swings to the bad eye, the light seems dimmer so both pupils enlarge. This observation is helpful because the neurologic exam may be otherwise unremarkable, without objective data to make a diagnosis or localize a lesion.

Although there are a number of causes of optic nerve dysfunction, the primary care physician needs to know only about two. These are optic neuritis (ON) and ischemic optic neuropathy. ON occurs in several disorders but most commonly in multiple sclerosis (MS), often as the initial feature.

ON may be painful or painless and its onset may be gradual or sudden. When it is painful, the pain is in the eye and may increase with eye movement. The globe and the fundus look normal if the inflammation is not near the optic head (where the nerve forms the optic disk). Pallor of the optic disk takes weeks to develop and, even when present, may be too subtle for a nonexpert to perceive. When the inflammation is at the nerve head, the disk is swollen and may contain hemorrhages. This therefore looks like unilateral papilledema but is actually papillitis, rather than papilledema, and thus does not signal increased intracranial pressure.

Since ON is a common feature of MS, the history should specifically cover the symptoms common in that disorder: gait dysfunction; bladder urgency, frequency, or incontinence; previous episodes of blurring or visual loss; episodes of diplopia; and family history of MS. Most MS patients are young or middle-aged adults, whereas the elderly hypertensive population develops ischemic optic nerve dysfunction. Other causes of ON are vasculitis, sarcoid, and postinfections or infections such as syphilis, tuberculosis, human immunodeficiency virus, cytomegalovirus, and herpes zoster.

Suspected cases of ON should be referred first to the ophthalmologist to confirm the diagnosis by excluding intraocular pathology and then to a neurologist to attempt diagnosis of the etiology of the ON. The first test of choice is magnetic resonance imaging (MRI) of the brain to look for demyelinated lesions. MRI of the optic nerves often shows the patch of active demyelination, which enhances with gadolinium. The nature of the MRI lesion, if limited to the optic nerve, however, is not helpful in making a diagnosis of the underlying condition.

Ischemic Disease

Ischemic problems affect either one eye or a visual field. Visual field problems that affect both eyes are always due to brain disease. Monocular visual problems are due to either retinal or optic nerve problems. A retinal problem may be evident on funduscopic examination, whereas an acute optic nerve problem usually does not reveal any abnormality other than an afferent defect. Altitudinal deficits, which affect the upper or lower half of vision in one eye, are always caused by retinal ischemia (Table 7.1).

Transient Monocular Blindness

Transient monocular blindness (TMB), also known as *amaurosis fugax*, is a transient ischemic attack (TIA) syndrome caused by inter-

Table 7.1.   Visual complaints and their localizations

Loss of vision in one eye (optic nerve or eye)
Field cut (brain)
Scotoma in one eye (retina)
Altitudinal field cut (retinal ischemia)
Double vision (eye muscle)
Hallucinations (eye, optic nerve, or brain)
Light flashes (retina)

rupted blood flow to the ophthalmic artery, a branch of the internal carotid. Patients describe the painless onset of a shade coming down or going up, a condition that can last up to 20 minutes without other symptoms. During the spell, which is rarely observed (I have examined one patient during a TMB spell in 20 years), the patient cannot see out of the affected eye and there is a markedly afferent pupillary deficit. The etiology of this syndrome often remains an enigma. On occasion, cholesterol emboli, called Hollenhorst's plaques, are seen in the retina, but these are usually not present and may be seen in patients without symptoms of TMB.

Although there is an increased association between TMB and hemispheric stroke, it is considerably less than the association between hemispheric TIA symptoms (hemiparesis, hemianesthesia, aphasia, and visual field cut) and strokes. There is a syndrome of recurrent TMB in young adults whose evaluation is negative for an explanation. They rarely go on to have a hemispheric stroke, although some do develop retinal infarction. TMB should be considered a cerebrovascular event and evaluated as a TIA. When carotid stenosis greater than 50% is found, an endarterectomy is indicated. When stenosis is less than 50%, other potential explanations must be considered. Evaluation of the aorta and heart for thrombus or right-to-left shunts may be required.

Ischemic Optic Neuropathy

Anterior ischemic optic neuropathy is a disease of older people. It falls into two categories. The more common form is idiopathic, associated with hypertension and other risk factors for cerebrovascular disease, and is most likely due to an atherosclerotic process. This condition is untreatable, does not resolve, and is basically a stroke of the optic nerve. About one-third of these patients develop disease in the other eye. Management is directed at reducing the various risk factors associated with vascular disease. The rarer form is due to giant cell (temporal) arteritis and is a medical emergency. Whereas the idiopathic anterior ischemic optic neuropathy usually occurs at the nerve head and causes disk swelling, ON from giant cell arteritis is retrobulbar and causes no acute disk change. The major distinguishing features, however, are the associated symptoms of temporal arteritis—namely, temporal tenderness, jaw claudication, fatigue, weight loss, malaise, low-grade fever, anemia, and a markedly elevated erythrocyte sedimentation rate (ESR). Only patients over age 60 should be suspected of having temporal arteritis. Since the second eye frequently goes blind and the process is never reversible, consideration of this diagnosis requires an immediate ESR test followed by treatment with methylprednisolone while awaiting the results of the ESR test. A normal or modestly elevated ESR rules out the diagnosis, and an ESR over 100 makes it more likely. The temporal artery biopsy can be obtained up to 1 week after the steroids have been started.

Field Cuts

Field cut is a nonspecific term that means a loss of vision in a region. Field cuts are called *homonymous* if they are the same in each eye or *incongruous* if different. Except for lesions of the optic chiasm, as occurs with pituitary tumors or with bilateral abnormalities of the optic nerves, field cuts are homonymous. Lesions affecting the optic chiasm interrupt the fibers from the medial aspects of both retinae, inducing loss of vision on the temporal side of each eye. Lesions in the hemispheres cause homonymous field cuts. The more posterior the lesion, the greater the congruity of the deficit. On bedside testing, however, one cannot expect to detect incongruities.

A homonymous hemianopia always indicates a hemispheric lesion, and its evaluation requires a brain imaging study and a neurologic referral.

Visual Hallucinations

Retinal tears cause a bright streak of light followed by an obscuration of the visual field in one eye. Bright flashes of light occur most commonly with migraines and retinal tears. Other causes such as occipital seizures are rare. Ischemic disorders do not cause bright flashes.

Formed Hallucinations

A benign syndrome of visual hallucinations commonly accompanies visual loss. These are called *release hallucinations* and may develop suddenly after acute onset of blindness or progress insidiously accompanying macular degeneration or severe cataracts. These are usually benign images and appear quite clearly, often with brilliant color and appearing only in the blind visual field. Patients usually have insight into the images' unreality, but if the images develop suddenly, then they are initially perceived as real. They are not associated with psychopathology, neuropathology, or dementia. They may resolve, stay the same, or worsen and they do not generally resolve with medications (such as antipsychotics or anticonvulsants). These are usually so mild that family members are unaware of their occurrence. The patient, realizing that everyone could think him or her crazy, never admits to the hallucinations. Occasionally, the visions are quite problematic. The hallucinations vary from unformed colors or lights to perfect images of people, animals, or objects. One unfortunate man I evaluated who was blind from macular degeneration had been "attacked" day and night for years by fast-moving lights that aimed for his head. Virtually every drug that crossed the blood-brain barrier and lidocaine injections of the optic nerves failed to reduce the severity.

HEARING LOSS AND TINNITUS

Deafness is a common problem, especially for the elderly, and goes hand in hand with tinnitus. Estimates on the prevalence vary, but more than 2.5 million Americans wear hearing aids and more than 25 million have significant hearing impairment. About half of children and about one-third of adults with hearing deficits acquire them based on heredity. Deafness is virtually never due to a central nervous system problem. This is presumably due to the auditory nerve's splitting twice on entering the brain stem to supply ipsilateral and contralateral input. Thus, bilateral lesions are required to impair hearing. Lesions of the acoustic nerve itself do, of course, produce deafness.

Deafness is caused by either sensorineural or conductive etiologies. Clinically these are distinguished by testing whether sound is better conducted through air or bone. With conductive loss, the bone acts as a better transmitter. Sensorineural loss diminishes sound via both media. General sensorineural deafness that occurs with aging reduces higher-pitched sounds, whereas conductive loss filters out lower-pitched sounds.

The type of sensorineural deafness that occurs with aging is called *presbycusis* and is thought to be due to neuronal degeneration. The other most common causes of sensorineural deafness are hereditary and mainly autosomal dominant. Although common sense would suggest that loud noises or explosions cause conductive problems with diminished low-frequency perception, they actually cause neural deficits with impaired high-pitch perception. This may be transient or sustained and is caused by damage to the cochlear hair cells.

Sudden deafness in one ear canal without vertigo is rare and may occur on a vascular basis from ischemia of the cochlea. Progressive deafness in one ear with episodic vertigo and tinnitus composes the triad of Ménière's disease.

Conductive hearing loss is non-neurologic in origin. Sudden deafness may be due to excess cerumen finally blocking a slightly open ear canal. Infections and trauma are the next most common causes. The examination should focus on the tympanic membrane.

Auditory Hallucinations

As with release hallucinations in blindness, some deaf people have
auditory hallucinations. These tend to occur in elderly patients with
long-standing deafness. The hallucinations occur in psychiatrically
normal individuals and tend to sound like music. They vary from
other everyday sounds and do not sound like sounds that occur with
tinnitus. As with release visual hallucinations of blindness, medications such as antipsychotics and anticonvulsants are not helpful.

Tinnitus

Although *tinnitus* means "ringing" in Latin, the term applies to a
large variety of sounds that originate in the ear. Some of these are
real sounds that emanate from other parts of the body, although most
are associated with abnormalities of hearing. Objective tinnitus may,
when circumstances are fortuitous, be heard by others. Palatal
myoclonus, a rare involuntary movement disorder of the palate,
causes a regular clicking sound similar to that of a ticking clock.
More common is a bruit due to turbulent blood flow in a large vessel
or an arteriovenous malformation in the neck or head. This type of
tinnitus is pulsatile and varies with the heartbeat. Pulsatile tinnitus is
also heard by the patient (not the examiner) with increased intracranial pressure, whether from pseudotumor cerebri or from an identified pathology such as a tumor.

   Most tinnitus occurs in association with hearing loss, but in
extremely quiet environments, most normal people experience some
degree of tinnitus. This is usually masked by the noise of our normal
environment. Tinnitus may be a ringing sound, musical tone, buzzing,
rushing, chirping, whooshing, or other similar noise. High-frequency
hearing loss is associated with a chirping sound and low frequency
with a whooshing sound. Conductive hearing loss (e.g., tympanic
membrane scarring) is associated with low-frequency tinnitus.

   A study of metabolic brain function in patients with tinnitus
showed marked changes in hearing pathways, implying an important

neurologic component to the tinnitus. This observation, however, cannot determine if the brain changes are secondary to ear-induced tinnitus or whether the tinnitus may have a neurogenic origin.

Regardless of the cause, unless it is due to an aspirin overdose (hence transient), tinnitus is almost impossible to treat. If the patient's tinnitus is pulsatile, the primary care physician should auscultate while having the patient facilitate the sound. If the sound is not audible, consideration of raised intracranial pressure should prompt a funduscopic examination to look for spontaneous venous pulsations and papilledema. In this setting, a neurologic consultation may be advisable, especially if a headache is present.

SMELL AND TASTE

Smell and taste are distinct neurologic functions yet are functionally closely related. It is commonly known that an unpalatable taste is best dealt with by holding one's nose to reduce the taste. A stuffed nose reduces enjoyment of pleasurable food or discomfort from poorly tasting fare. Yet, innervation is quite distinct. Smell is subserved by the first (olfactory) nerve that innervates the receptors in the upper nose. Taste is perceived by cranial nerves V, VII, IX, and X. Within the brain, there is widespread distribution of impulses through which smell modifies taste. The smell perception network is phylogenetically old and is closely related to structures involved in emotions and memory.

Disorders of smell and taste are estimated to affect 1–25% of Americans, but such disorders are uncommonly brought to medical attention. The most common smell complaint is anosmia or hyposmia, which is usually the result of a nasal or sinus problem. Cigarette smoking and other toxins are contributory. Most smell problems are conductive problems. Nasal polyps, upper respiratory infections, and allergies are the usual culprits, and symptom severity varies with the degree of obstruction. Smell may also be lost with viral infections, presumably directly affecting the chemoreceptors. The nasal epithelium is considered a potential route of entry for some virus infections, suggesting that the virus may directly affect the receptor. Neurologic causes of smell dysfunction are rare, aside from head trauma. Estimates that 5% of head trauma patients suffer anosmia are in the literature, but how severe this head trauma must be is unclear. The development of anosmia after a significant head injury, however, should be considered posttraumatic and carries a poor prognosis for recovery of smell. Patients frequently do not appreciate the loss at first but become very bothered by it later.

Deficiencies of odor perception are common in both Parkinson's disease and Alzheimer's disease, but these rarely occur at the symptomatic level. It would be extraordinary for a patient with either disease to present with a complaint related to smell.

Rarely, patients with MS may have deficiencies of odor perception. Hallucinated smells are notable auras of some psychomotor seizures. These are usually foul smells and last for seconds before the motor component of the seizure develops.

Most patients with taste loss actually have problems with odor perception and not that of taste. Certain medications, zinc deficiency, cigarette smoking, throat and tongue radiation for cancer, chemotherapy, and opportunistic infections like monilia, however, may damage the epithelial lining of the tongue and throat and destroy the chemoreceptors. Sinusitis or postnasal drip causes a constant bad taste. Altered taste sensation, called *dysgeusia*, almost always induces a bad taste and often has no identifiable explanation.

Aside from head trauma, neurologic explanations for taste and smell problems are rare. Patients with these problems should be referred to otolaryngologists or taste and smell centers if a review of medications and history does not yield an answer.

CLINICAL PEARLS

- Blurred vision of neurologic origin is usually due to diplopia so mild that the images are too close to be recognized as separate. Closing either eye resolves the blurring.

- Optic nerve dysfunction may cause blurring, in which case vision in only the affected eye is blurred. This cannot be corrected with lenses.
- Diplopia with one eye (while the other is closed) is either due to isolated eye disease or is psychogenic.
- Visual hallucinations, formed or unformed, may occur with loss of vision in any part of the visual path.
- Auditory hallucinations may accompany deafness.
- Visual loss from temporal arteritis is an emergency requiring steroids.
- Most taste abnormalities are due to smell dysfunction.
- Blurred vision due to extraocular muscle weakness resolves when either eye is closed.
- Impaired vision in one eye is due to optic nerve or eye disease, not brain disease.
- Head trauma frequently causes smell and therefore taste dysfunction.

8

Transient Ischemic Attack and Stroke

Stroke is a common, often devastating event whose frequency increases with age. It is the third leading cause of death in the United States after cardiovascular disease and cancer. It is the leading cause of neurologic morbidity and the single most common neurologic reason for hospitalization. Every physician who cares for adult patients in any capacity sees patients with cerebrovascular disease (CVD). Neurology training, historically hospital-founded, has been so heavily based on stroke-related admissions that the famous neurologist C. Miller Fisher noted that neurologists learn their discipline "stroke by stroke."

As our understanding of strokes increases, it has become evident that strokes are often preventable and that stroke rates are decreased with the implementation of better recognition and treatment of hypertension, heart diseases, hyperlipidemia, and cigarette addiction. Despite decades of endarterectomies, proof has emerged only recently that in some situations, carotid endarterectomy does reduce stroke risk. Antiplatelet agents have shown definite, albeit small, benefit in reducing stroke risk. And for the first time, thrombolytic therapy, if used within 3 hours, has been shown to reduce stroke deficit. This latter finding has translated into a concerted push by the neurologic community to alert patients to the importance of recognizing stroke symptoms at their onset and seeking medical attention as soon as possible. This has led to catchy slogans to spread the news: a stroke is now described as a "brain attack," and there are other catch phrases such as "time is brain" and "a brain is a terrible thing to waste."

This excitement reflects a newly found sense of optimism. Although stroke incidence has declined dramatically over the past 4 decades, stroke outcome is still poor. Almost one-fourth of stroke victims die and an additional 15–30% go to nursing homes. With thrombolytic therapy there is hope that these numbers can also be improved.

The topic of CVD can be approached from two perspectives: physiologic and phenomenologic. The latter has strong implications for the former because phenomenology leads to localization that helps determine treatment.

Strokes come in two and one-half types. Either blood flow is inadequate, leading to neuronal death from ischemia, or a blood vessel ruptures, resulting in free blood. The former type of stroke is called an *infarct* and the latter a *hemorrhage*. The "half" variety of stroke has characteristics of both—namely, an infarct with blood. Most infarcts do not contain blood and are called *bland infarcts*. In some cases, probably more common with embolic occlusions, infarction is followed by restoration of blood flow, typically after an embolus dissolves. The blood flows through friable tissue, resulting in extravasation. Most hemorrhagic infarcts are largely bland, with regions of purpuric-like blood collections. Some, however, are largely blood clots in the middle of a larger infarcted region.

A transient ischemic attack (TIA) is a temporary neurologic dysfunction occurring in a vascular distribution, persisting for under 24 hours and leaving no neurologic residua and no alteration on brain imaging. In other words, the episode lasts under 24 hours and there is no infarcted tissue.

The mechanisms underlying stroke are not fully understood, and strokes in different regions of the brain appear to have different pathophysiologies. Certainly any part of the brain is subject to embolic infarction. A chunk of something is knocked off its resting place by flowing blood and clogs a distal artery. Generally the embolus is then broken down by enzymes in the blood, but by the time this is complete and blood flow is restored, some tissue has infarcted.

The embolus arises in the heart (due to wall dyskinesis, atrial enlargement, or valvular disease), the large arteries (ascending aorta, carotid, or vertebral arteries), or, rarely, on the venous side and then passes to the arterial side via a patent foramen ovale. The embolus may be arteriosclerotic debris with cholesterol crystals, platelet and fibrin deposits, bacterial and fibrin platelet globs in endocarditis, or frank blood clots. Emboli from the heart, aorta, and carotid tend to enter the internal carotid, then middle cerebral artery territory due to the large volume of blood flowing to this vessel and the geometry favoring a "straight shoot."

It is easy to understand how emboli cause strokes. It is less comprehensible why blood flow impairment in the carotid should cause focal hemispheric symptoms, but this clearly occurs. Stroke risk has been correlated with carotid stenosis and occlusion. It has not yet been correlated with the degree of ulceration in carotid plaques, although this is a potential source of emboli. Increasing blood flow by removing stenosis reduces stroke risk in patients who have had TIAs or strokes. There are occasional patients in whom low blood pressure causes focal symptoms, but this is rare. A famous British study explored this possibility by examining a large group of patients with TIAs. Patients had their autonomic nervous system paralyzed and then were laid on tilt tables. The table was rotated to the upright position and blood pressure fell. Only a few of these patients experienced TIAs. The others fainted. Fortunately for all involved, no one had a stroke. Common sense, if not the Helsinki accords, keeps this study from being replicated, but its outcome parallels clinical experience. Yet, if all TIAs and most strokes were embolic in origin, the partly random nature of blood flow implies TIA clinical phenomena should be somewhat random, which is not the case. Most TIAs are rather stereotypic for each patient.

Strokes in the anterior (internal carotid, middle, and anterior cerebral arteries) and posterior (vertebral, basilar, and posterior cerebral arteries) circulations have different pathophysiologic mechanisms. Posterior circulation strokes are more commonly due to thrombus than anterior circulation strokes. Why this is the case is unexplained.

In addition, vertebral-basilar strokes are often due to thrombotic occlusions at some distance proximal to the infarcted region. For example, in a famous study of the Wallenberg syndrome (posterior inferior cerebellar artery [PICA] occlusion), most cases had thrombus in the vertebral artery and not the PICA, which was patent.

Lacunar infarcts are spherical holes with a diameter measured in millimeters that occur as the result of slowly progressive occlusion of penetrating arterioles by a process called *lipohyalinosis*. This describes the pathologic material that accumulates in the vessel walls. Lacunar infarcts generally are associated with hypertension, but not always. There are a variety of lacunar syndromes. The infarcts usually are located in the internal capsule, thalamus, or basal ganglia. Although the pathologic process is slowly progressive, the stroke develops suddenly like other strokes and may be preceded by TIAs.

RISK FACTORS

The single greatest risk factor for stroke is previous CVD, particularly previous stroke or TIA. Most stroke risk factors are closely related to cardiovascular risk factors, with hypertension and diabetes being foremost. Virtually all heart disorders predispose to stroke, but certain ones deserve special attention. Isolated atrial fibrillation increases stroke risk by a factor of 4, but atrial fibrillation with mitral valve disease, as is typical of rheumatic heart disease, increases risk by a factor of 14. Until recently there were no data to determine whether paroxysmal atrial fibrillation poses an equal, reduced, or greater risk than chronic fibrillation. Data suggest they have comparable risk, but factors such as frequency of rhythm changes, atrial size, and etiology of the atrial fibrillation are important. Ventricular hypokinesis leads to cardioembolic disease, with anterior wall involvement causing the greatest risk. Recognition of this fact led to the current recommendation of heparinization of all patients with anterior wall myocardial infarcts. Cardiomyopathies, whether due to inflammation or valvular or ischemic disease, all increase cardioembolic risk and thus the risk of stroke. Coronary artery disease (CAD) is highly associated with stroke risk, even in the absence of a myocardial infarction. CAD is not necessarily an etiology for stroke but simply a marker for vascular disease, much more so than peripheral vascular disease. Less important risk factors include cigarette smoking and hyperlipidemia.

CLINICAL ASPECTS

Most strokes are sudden in onset, although some may have a stuttering progression. Often patients awaken in the morning unaware that they have suffered a stroke during sleep until they try to get out of bed.

Infarcts are not usually associated with symptoms other than the neurologic deficit. That is, most strokes are not associated with significant headache or nausea. Except for brain stem strokes, loss of consciousness is rarely a feature of either stroke or TIA. Having noted this, which is certainly true for most strokes, I point out that brain hemorrhages and brain stem infarcts are often associated with headache or nausea.

TIAs classically last about 20 minutes. A TIA of the ophthalmic artery or of the circulation to the optic nerve is often called *amaurosis fugax* ("fleeting blindness") but in neurologic jargon has come to be called *transient monocular blindness* (TMB). Although symptomatic of CVD, it has a more benign prognosis than other TIA syndromes. The patient describes a curtain rapidly descending. There is a loss of vision but not blackness. Because the abnormality is in the eye or optic nerve and not the brain, the blindness is monocular rather than a field cut, which patients frequently mistake for loss of vision on one side. TMB is associated with carotid stenosis and stroke but much less so than brain TIAs.

TIAs precede infarcts but not hemorrhages in 20–40% of cases. This percentage varies with the series, reflecting either population differences (different ethnic populations, in fact, have different stroke profiles) or differences in data acquisition. Most stroke patients have not had TIAs. The risk of stroke after a TIA is only about 20% by 5 years. This means that a TIA is not a cataclysmic event. Most patients do not have an imminent stroke. Many of these patients have myocardial infarctions too. Aside from TMB, the common TIA syndromes are weakness or sensory loss on one side or in one limb and difficulty with speech due either to dysarthria or aphasia. Posterior circulation TIAs causing ataxia or diplopia are far less common. TIAs rarely cause loss of consciousness, light headedness, or vertigo in the absence of other neurologic symptoms. (These issues are discussed in greater detail below.)

Brain hemorrhages are either parenchymal (into the brain) or subarachnoid. The latter are aneurysmal bleeds and not common. Patients with ruptured (berry) aneurysms bleed into the spinal fluid and present with sudden coma or severe headache, usually without focal symptoms. Intraparenchymal hemorrhages are usually due to one of two conditions: hypertensive hemorrhages or lobar hemorrhages. Hypertensive hemorrhages are due to Charcot-Bouchard aneurysms (small arteriolar aneurysms) that burst. These occur in the same locations as lacunar infarcts, also associated with chronic hypertension: in the basal ganglia, thalamus, internal capsule, cerebellum, and pons. In the nonhypertensive elderly, the most common cause for intraparenchymal hemorrhage is amyloid angiopathy, a condition not associated with systemic amyloid. This condition is also called *congophilic angiopathy* due to its histologic staining characteristics. The location of these hemorrhages is at the cortical white matter junction rather than deep in the hemisphere, as occurs with hypertensive hemorrhage. The prognosis for recovery from each event is generally better with amyloid angiopathic hemorrhages, which are usually also called *lobar hemorrhages* due to their restriction to a single brain lobe, but the long-term prognosis is not good because more hemorrhages typically occur and there is no known method to reduce risk.

STROKE SYNDROMES

Although there are a huge number of stroke syndromes, including the eponymic brain stem stroke syndromes of the nineteenth century (Weber, Benedikt, Millard-Gubler, Foville, Wallenburg), there are really

Table 8.1.   Common stroke phenomenology

Lacunes: pure weakness or pure sensory loss
Anterior cerebral artery: leg weakness and numbness ± mental changes
Middle cerebral artery: aphasia or agnosias ± gaze deviation ± field cut or
    face and arm weakness > leg weakness or mild sensory loss
Brain stem: crossed findings or ataxia or eye movement or pupil dysfunction

only a handful of stroke syndromes that any primary care physician
(PCP) should know. Infarcts are usually described by the vascular territory affected. The most common stroke syndromes are lacunes and
large-vessel strokes occurring in the distribution of the anterior, middle,
or posterior cerebral arteries or in the vertebral-basilar system. We
divide these into *anterior*, meaning the anterior and middle cerebral
arteries that arise from the internal carotid, and *posterior*, referring to
the vessels arising from the vertebral and basilar arteries (Table 8.1).

Anterior Circulation Strokes

Middle Cerebral Artery Strokes

Middle cerebral artery strokes are the most common large-vessel
hemispheric strokes. The mental manifestations vary with the side of
the brain affected, but the other findings are independent of side. With
language-dominant hemisphere involvement (usually the left), the
patient is aphasic. Most aphasias do not fit a classic pattern early on
(i.e., Broca's, Wernicke's, conduction, etc.) and instead evolve into the
variously catalogued aphasia types over months. In a crude fashion,
aphasia is categorized by the ability to produce words and by the
degree of retained comprehension. Global aphasia means destroyed
language function (nothing comes in or out). With a nondominant
hemisphere stroke, the major mental abnormality is neglect and frequently denial. Patients are unaware of the left side of space and the
left side of their body. They lose insight into their illness and deny any
disability. Usually the more severe the infarct, the better these patients

feel. They do not perceive weakness, sensory loss, or any problem at all, even if they know at some intellectual level that they have had a stroke. These patients have difficulty with rehabilitation because they cannot be trained to deal with a problem they do not believe they have. In contrast to psychiatric disorders, these mental abnormalities are due to a failure to recognize, rather than a suppression of recognition.

The cranial nerve abnormalities with middle cerebral artery strokes may include gaze deviation, with the eyes deviated to the side of the lesion (away from the weakness), and a contralateral homonymous field cut. Facial weakness, decreased shoulder shrug, and tongue deviation are standard.

The motor examination reveals weakness of arm and leg. Unless the stroke is massive, the face and arm are more affected than the leg. The sensory deficit is in the same distribution as the weakness but is a less prominent symptom. Patients still perceive on the affected side, but they lose some discriminatory capabilities. Sharp is perceived as duller on the affected side. Graphesthesia and two-point discrimination are reduced. The patient can walk if the affected leg is not paralyzed, but the affected leg is stiff, with diminished knee flexion, and the affected arm swings less.

Anterior Cerebral Artery Strokes

Anterior cerebral artery strokes are uncommon despite the fact that both the anterior and middle cerebral arteries are branches of the internal carotid. The clinical syndrome is a relatively isolated contralateral leg weakness and numbness. There may or may not be arm weakness, physical changes, or mental changes, including apraxia, mutism, and mental slowness.

Lacunar Strokes

Lacunes occur in the internal capsule, thalamus, basal ganglia, and pons. These locations are the same as those in which hypertensive hemorrhages occur, presumably because arterioles in these regions are more susceptible to changes induced by longstanding hypertension.

The most common lacunar syndrome is a *pure motor stroke*. It is due to an infarct in the internal capsule. There are no mental status changes with the first few lacunes. The cranial nerve changes affect the face and possibly cause shoulder shrug and tongue weakness. The arm or leg may also be affected. The involvement of face, arm, and leg, approximately equally, are the classic lacunes with no other neurologic change. It has become clear that variable combinations of face, arm, or leg involvement are possible with strategically placed lacunes.

The second most common syndrome is a *pure sensory stroke*, which usually splits midline and thus sometimes is misinterpreted as a functional, nonphysiologic abnormality.

There are, in addition to the above, over 20 other lacunar syndromes. Pure sensory stroke and especially pure motor stroke occur so frequently as to be required knowledge. The others are rare enough to be considered arcane.

Posterior Circulation Strokes

Recognition of ischemic events in the vertebral-basilar distribution is important because the carotids are not involved and therefore do not need to be studied. Surgery is not an option.

Posterior circulation strokes are recognizable by one or more of four syndromes: crossed findings, cerebellar ataxia, pupillary dysfunction, or eye movement abnormalities (excluding conjugate gaze deviation).

The principle of *crossed findings* rests on the observation that the corticospinal tract controlling voluntary movements crosses in the lower brain stem, and the spinothalamic tract, which delivers most sensory information to the brain, crosses sides within the spinal cord. An infarct in the brain stem causes an abnormality of the cranial nerves on the same side at the level of the stroke but may interrupt the passing corticospinal or sensory pathways that have crossed at a lower level. This causes an interruption of function of the ipsilateral cranial nerve but affects the opposite side of the body below the cranial nerve malfunction. One side of the face is affected while the other side of the body is affected. Thus the stroke causes "crossed" findings.

Cerebellar ataxia, like so much of neurologic phenomenology, is easier to recognize than to describe. There are no good definitions of ataxia that I have seen. Basically, one or more limbs become very clumsy and poorly coordinated without any loss of strength. It can be difficult to distinguish ataxia from corticospinal tract damage that fails to induce weakness but does cause clumsiness. Midline cerebellar lesions cause isolated gait ataxia. The legs are not ataxic while the patient is seated or lying in bed; only walking brings the ataxia out.

Brain stem lesions may affect the pupils, causing an oval shape, dilatation, or failure to react (midbrain). One may instead see a pinpoint pupil (pons) or Horner's syndrome. Dysconjugate gaze is always the result of a brain stem lesion's causing a cranial neuropathy.

One other aspect of brain stem stroke bears mentioning. Because the basilar artery is unpaired and gives rise to the two posterior cerebral arteries, a single lesion in the basilar artery may cause bilateral infarcts. Anterior circulation strokes, however, cause only unilateral signs and symptoms. A single basilar artery stroke may cause crossed findings as noted before or bilateral abnormalities—for example, quadriparesis or bilateral blindness.

HEMORRHAGES

Intraparenchymal hemorrhages may not occur in single vascular territories. When a hemorrhage is in the territory of what would otherwise be a typical infarct, one must strongly consider the diagnosis of hemorrhagic infarct. Hypertensive hemorrhages are generally deep, causing a hemiparesis that may look clinically like a lacunar infarct. Lobar hemorrhages are near the surface, often causing relatively isolated limb weakness or visual loss.

Subarachnoid hemorrhage is caused by spontaneous rupture of a berry aneurysm. These are usually located at the bifurcation of the vessels in the circle of Willis at the base of the brain. These vessels are in the skull but outside of the brain. When the aneurysm ruptures, a small volume of blood, perhaps 10 ml or less, suddenly shoots out of the artery under systolic blood pressure. This sudden, high-pressure injection of blood causes an effect similar to several hammers hitting the head at the same time from all directions. The patient experiences the sudden onset of the worst headache ever experienced and frequently collapses. Focal symptoms are uncommon early on. If the aneurysm is pointing upward, however, the jet of blood can dissect into the brain and cause focal signs. Often the patient is stuporous or comatose, which carries a worse prognosis. Focal symptoms may arise days later due to delayed arterial spasm. Symptomatic hydrocephalus with decreased consciousness also occurs as delayed phenomena.

EVALUATION AND TREATMENT

The evaluation of CVD makes sense only if it alters management. Treatment of CVD, except in the first 3 hours, is prophylactic only. At this time the treatment decisions are limited to antiplatelet agents, anticoagulation, endarterectomy, blood pressure control, or nothing. If the patient is not a surgical candidate, then there is little, if any, role for a carotid ultrasound. A computed tomography (CT) scan is usually sufficient. Brain imaging accomplishes two things. The first is exclusion of other mechanisms for the TIA because about 10% of presumed TIAs are due to other lesions such as tumors, arteriovenous malformations, or brain hemorrhages. Imaging also detects clinically silent strokes that may implicate unknown disease on the other side or strokes in several vascular territories, implying a possible cardiac or aortic source. Because studies have convincingly demonstrated that endarterectomies on symptomatic carotid stenosis of 70% or more reduce the incidence of stroke (if the surgeon has a morbidity rate of less than 5%), the treatment of choice for 50–99% stenosis is an endarterectomy. When the carotid is completely blocked, endarterectomy is not possible because the clot propagates up into the skull and becomes unresectable. Posterior circulation strokes may require magnetic resonance imaging (MRI) to rule out a tumor or to identify and localize the process. Carotid studies are pointless for evaluating vertebrobasilar symptoms.

Carotid duplex studies measure flow velocity and also provide an image of the blood vessels. However, these studies are not as accurate as standard angiography, and accuracy varies from lab to lab. The "gold standard" for assessing stenosis remains the standard angiogram. Magnetic resonance angiography (MRA) exaggerates the degree of stenosis. Most, but not all, surgeons want a standard angiogram before surgery. As magnetic resonance techniques improve, MRA will undoubtedly supplant conventional angiography.

Acute strokes are treatable if the stroke is a bland infarct caught within 3 hours of onset. In this uncommon situation, tissue plasminogen activator (t-PA) has been shown to reduce stroke deficit. But the t-PA must be given within 3 hours of onset and the brain image must demonstrate no developing large acute infarct and no blood. Because t-PA actually increases death rate in stroke patients and bleeding problems in general, the decision to give t-PA should be made by experienced clinicians. Bell's palsies, peripheral nerve lesions, multiple sclerosis, focal seizures, and spinal cord problems are frequently misdiagnosed as strokes.

If a patient wakes up with a new deficit, t-PA should not be given because the time of onset of the stroke is unknown and may have exceeded the allowed time frame. The reason for being so scrupulous about stroke-onset time is that trials of t-PA and other "clot busters" used after 3 hours of onset led to more complications and no significant improvement compared to untreated patients. Thus, delayed treatment is worse than no treatment.

The use of heparin in acute stroke is unresolved. I typically recommend its use early on if the stroke appears to be "incomplete" in the sense that it could worsen. The risk of bleeding is small. For anterior circulation strokes, I switch to aspirin after about 2 days. For posterior circulation strokes, I recommend warfarin sodium (Coumadin) for 30 days. This approach is as good as any, but it is not justified by data. Few data exist on management of the acute stroke. Steroids are of no benefit at any time.

STROKE OUTCOMES

Management of the acute stroke syndrome is usually performed either by the PCP, neurologist, or both. Long-term management, however, almost always is the province of the PCP, with occasional input by the neurologist. It is therefore helpful to the PCP in particular to know about short-term and long-term prognoses.

Short-Term Outcome

At the onset of a stroke, few factors are reliable predictors of outcome. Acute CT changes seen early always predict worse outcome. Brain hemorrhages obviously are not TIAs and do not resolve in a few hours. Stupor and coma are always grim prognostic factors unless due to systemic infections such as urinary tract infection or pneumonia, or to a postseizure state.

Most stroke recovery occurs early, leading to the common sense observation that the longer a deficit lasts, the less likely it is to resolve. Other prognostic observations can also be made with common sense. The greater the age, the less resilient the brain's recuperative powers. The presence of complicating features such as infection, myocardial infarct, and renal failure worsens the outcome.

Two general facts worth citing to patient and family early on, because they carry hope, are that motor recovery is thought to continue for 3 months before reaching a plateau, and language and mental function are thought to reach a plateau only by 6 months. Thus, even with a severe deficit at the time of hospital discharge 3 or 4 days after the stroke, there is still a lot of time for functionally important recovery.

Gaze deviation, for unknown reason, always resolves and does so within the first 3 days in most cases. Stupor, if present early, is a bad prognostic sign but resolves within a few days if the patient survives.

Stupor that develops during days 3–5 may represent cerebral edema, which is a very bad sign because it suggests brain herniation.

Long-Term Outcome

Prognosis After First Stroke

In a 1998 report from the Mayo Clinic, about 7% of first-stroke patients died in the first week, 14% within a month, 27% at 1 year, and 53% by 5 years. This does not take into account the various stroke risk factors and represents an overall synopsis. Age, heart disease (heart failure, ischemic heart disease, and atrial fibrillation), and recurrent stroke were the major risk factors for early death. The risk of a second stroke was 12% at 1 year and 29% by 5 years.

Functional Recovery

In a prospective British study, 88% of stroke patients had a hemiparesis at the onset. By 1 month, 26% had no impairment and 39% were only mildly affected. By 6 months, 39% had no impairment and 36% had mild impairment. Mild hemiparesis at onset resulted in complete recovery 10 times more often than severe weakness at onset.

Arm function recovered to full use in 79% of those with mild weakness but only 18% in those with severe weakness at presentation. No hand movement at 2 weeks presaged a poor recovery.

In another prospective study involving 800 patients, 51% were unable to walk at onset. All received extensive rehabilitation. Only one-third of these patients were then able to walk independently. Less than one-fourth of patients admitted with mild to moderate leg weakness could later walk 150 feet independently. With leg paralysis, the rate was considerably worse. Physical therapy is very helpful for improving functional recovery. Speech and cognitive therapies, while given, have not been clearly shown to be beneficial.

About half of aphasics recover good language function, but other cognitive skills are differentially affected. Although dementia is rarely caused by a single stroke, the incidence of dementia is almost 10 times greater within 1 year of a stroke than in an age-matched population. Right hemisphere deficits, such as denial and neglect, sensory extinction, and anosognosia, that present such interesting phenomenology that they are often used as teaching cases and form the subject of essays by Oliver Sacks, usually resolve within 6 months.

The mechanisms of recovery are complex and poorly understood. Early recovery is due to damaged but not infarcted parts of the brain recovering. Neurologists and radiologists talk of the *ischemic penumbra*, a region of the brain damaged, but not necessarily irreversibly, by ischemia. The ischemic penumbra has inspired intense research to devise drugs that keep damaged, but not yet dead, regions from actually dying.

Long-term recovery is correlated with a number of factors. There is some degree of brain plasticity, proved in both animals and humans undergoing brain mapping, that varies with age, baseline brain function, and the part of the brain affected. However, psychologic states such as mood and motivation, family support, and level of education are important factors in long-term rehabilitation. Depression is common but treatable. Failure to recognize it always impedes recovery.

CLINICAL PEARLS

- Anterior circulation strokes rarely cause loss of consciousness.
- Transient episodes of loss of consciousness or lightheadedness should not be considered TIAs unless focal neurologic symptoms were also present.
- Cerebellar hemorrhages should be evaluated by a neurosurgeon if the patient is not comatose more than a few minutes. By the time the patient has been in coma for an hour, return of brain stem function is unlikely when the clot is removed.
- Posterior circulation cerebrovascular symptoms should not be evaluated with carotid ultrasound.
- All young patients and some older patients with unexplained stroke should have a bubble study with transesophageal cardiac echocardiography to evaluate the possibility of a patent foramen ovale (right to left shunt).

Table 8.2.   Prophylaxis against anterior circulation strokes

1. Carotid endarterectomy if stenosis > 50% in symptomatic vessel
2. Aspirin, 1–4 tablets/day
3. Ticlopidine or clopidigrel for aspirin failures (clopidigrel is easier to use)

- Brain stem strokes, unlike hemispheric strokes, may progress slowly over days, simulating a neoplasm (both clinically and by CT appearance). Hemispheric strokes may progress suddenly in stages but do so only over the first day or two.
- Hypertensive and amyloid angiopathic brain hemorrhages do not rebleed in the first few weeks unless a coagulation deficit is present.
- Stroke patients without cardiac abnormalities do not require an echocardiogram.
- After a carotid endarterectomy, a patient should remain on aspirin for life.
- After a massive infarct, only an antiplatelet drug is indicated, not endarterectomy.
- Patients with atrial fibrillation, regardless of age, should be treated with warfarin sodium (Coumadin) if their risk of injury on the drug is not so high that it outweighs the risk of a stroke (e.g., having active epilepsy).
- Ischemia usually causes negative phenomena, whereas seizures generally cause positive phenomena. Thus, strokes usually cause weakness or numbness (a "dead" or "wooden" sensation). Seizures typically cause jerking, stiffness, tingling, burning, or other uncomfortable sensations.
- Every person older than age 50 should take a small dose of aspirin daily to reduce stroke risk (Table 8.2).
- Fever is almost never of central nervous system origin. Stroke patients with fever are infected. Patients with spinal cord transections, however, have severe thermoregulatory problems and may have hyperthermia without infection (although this must be evaluated).

9

Trauma

The primary care physician (PCP) is involved in the assessment of minor head injury only. The question of what constitutes minor versus severe is usually straightforward. PCPs are typically involved with management of head trauma that causes either brief or no loss of consciousness.

CONCUSSION

The definition of *concussion* has been somewhat flexible. Typically, concussion had been defined as a syndrome of loss of consciousness or memory due to head injury. The American Academy of Neurology (AAN), however, has adopted a broader definition that accepts an immediate or slightly delayed confusional or amnestic syndrome after head trauma as a concussion. Severity of concussion can be identified by a series of grades. Grade 1 concussion has no loss of consciousness and an amnestic or confusional syndrome resolving within 15 minutes. Grade 2 concussion is the same as grade 1 but lasts longer than 15 minutes. Grade 3 concussion involves any loss of consciousness regardless of the duration or speed of recovery.

When trauma has just occurred, patients are often taken to the emergency room (ER) or to the PCP's office. Because ER visits for head trauma are so common and the possible choices for management vary so much in cost, various options have been studied for both cost and outcome. Before the era of computed tomography (CT) scans, patients had a skull x-ray and were either admitted for observation or sent home with a "head sheet," which was a list of instructions for observing for potential danger signals: excessive sleepiness, vomiting, confusion, and unequal pupils. The advent of CT made it possible to image the brain to exclude brain hematomas and contusions and therefore more confidently predict who might require neurosurgical intervention. The use of CT is expensive, however, and at large, busy centers where trauma is common, it creates potential delays in providing care.

For the PCP there are basically three types of head trauma patients: the acute patient, who comes to the office shortly after the event; the patient who reports an event that occurred in the past few days or weeks; and the "high-risk" patient, who is either elderly or has a bleeding diathesis.

The patient who had a grade 1 or 2 concussion the day of the evaluation requires only a neurologic examination. The presence of any neurologic sign, including even mild confusion, merits a brain CT scan. If the concussion induced loss of consciousness or amnesia, a CT scan of the brain, including "bone windows" for assessing the skull's integrity, should be obtained. In both prospective and retrospective studies it is clear that only a very small minority of healthy patients with minor head injuries go on to develop neurological problems and virtually all of these had suffered skull fractures. It is likely that the skull fracture is simply a marker for the severity of the impact and has no implications on its own except in critical locations. Those that cross the middle meningeal groove may cause a life-threatening epidural hematoma (see "Epidural Hematoma," below), and those at the base of the skull may cause a cerebrospinal fluid (CSF) leak. CSF leaks are best detected by an enhanced brain CT that shows air (very dark regions) in the head. This may not be present early on, but when these regions are found, the patient requires a neurosurgical evaluation.

The AAN has developed guidelines for the resumption of sporting activities after concussions (Table 9.1).

Because some problems develop hours after the head trauma, instructions should be given to a reliable family member or friend to look for signs of increased intracranial pressure. These are primarily decreased alertness, vomiting, or any new neurologic aberration.

Table 9.1.   Guidelines for returning to athletics after concussion[a]

Type of concussion	Time before returning
Grade 1[b]	Same day upon returning to normal
Repeated grade 1	1 wk
Grade 2[c]	1 wk
Repeated grade 2	2 wks
Grade 3[d] (brief)	1 wk
Grade 3 (mins)	2 wks
Repeated grade 3	1 mo or longer

[a]Recommendations of American Academy of Neurology, 1997.
[b]Grade 1: No loss of consciousness. Amnesia or confusion lasts under 15 minutes.
[c]Grade 2: No loss of consciousness. Amnesia or confusion lasts over 15 minutes.
[d]Grade 3: Loss of consciousness of any duration.

Head trauma in the elderly and in those with a bleeding diathesis generally requires a brain CT. Coagulation abnormalities must be reversed if blood is seen on the CT. Subdural hematomas in the elderly are generally not emergency conditions unless the patient is deteriorating. It must be noted that as a result of atrophy, the elderly are subject to subdural hematomas with only minimal trauma. These are often managed conservatively, with observation only and serial scans. This decision should be made by a neurologist or neurosurgeon.

CT is a much more sensitive and useful tool for evaluating trauma than magnetic resonance imaging (MRI). The CT shows acute blood in the subarachnoid space as well as the brain, subdural, and epidural spaces. An MRI is actually less sensitive and more difficult to interpret for trauma.

After minor head trauma, most patients recover to normal. Severe head injury causes a constellation of changes that vary with the severity. An important general principle after severe head injury in which coma lasting hours or longer occurs is that recovery is far better than recovery from a coma due to nontraumatic causes. Even patients with few brain stem reflexes at coma onset may walk out of the hospital months later. Therefore, one cannot prognosticate after head trauma as early as one can after cardiac arrest, in which recovery is unlikely if the patient is still comatose even 1 day later.

After minor concussive injuries, two distinct problems may occur. One is postconcussive syndrome and the other is post-traumatic seizure.

Postconcussive Syndrome

Postconcussive syndrome has a large set of badly defined symptoms. What is most striking is that the same set of complaints occurs worldwide with minor head injuries. The most common symptoms are headache, disequilibrium, diminished attention, and impaired memory. The headache is of variable severity and is usually holoacranial but may either be localized or most severe at the point of impact. The pain is usually constant and aching. It shares many attributes with the pain of tension headaches, but throbbing and stabbing pains are also described. These headaches are the most common sequelae of head injury bringing the patient to the neurologist's attention. The sense of disequilibrium is often described as dizziness, but the term *dizzy*, which does not usually connote any sense of true vertigo, is a more diffuse term in this disorder. Patients feel a sense of mental fogginess, as if their thinking is mildly unclear and uncertain. Patients also have a mild decrease in their reliance on their motor prowess. Thus, the patient feels both physically and cognitively impaired. Some patients also develop a degree of emotional unsteadiness, as if their coping skills are mildly impaired in social situations, particularly those required in complex situations. My own experience with these patients, particularly in high-functioning students, is that impaired concentration is the largest problem. At times this is partly due to headaches, but not always. Impaired concentration, of course, always leads to reduced ability to lay down new memory traces, which impairs learning and diminishes school performance.

The duration of the postconcussive syndrome varies with the severity of impact, the personality of the subject, and the presence of litigation. Many of the symptoms of depression and anxiety may also be present or may be the primary problems. Reassurance is the most important treatment. Once serious problems, such as subdural hematomas, have been excluded, the headache should be addressed as a

Table 9.2.   Epidural hematoma

Cause: rupture of the middle meningeal artery due to fracture of
   temporal bone
Course: coma followed by regained consciousness for a few minutes
   and then coma
Management: immediate (emergency room) evacuation of blood clot

tension-type headache. Other aspects are treatable only by time, psy-chotherapy, or antidepressants, if appropriate. Generally symptoms improve or resolve by 6 months.

Post-Traumatic Seizures

Post-traumatic seizures occurring within the first 7 days of a concus-sion are not considered prognostic of post-traumatic epilepsy, whereas those occurring after 7 days are. The report of a seizure at the time of the head trauma should not be interpreted as an ominous sign. In fact, these patients should not be placed on anticonvulsants unless they have had additional seizures. By 6 months after the head injury, half the patients destined to have seizures have had them. By 1 year, only 25% of those who have seizures have not already had one.

Post-traumatic seizures are managed according to the same prin-ciples as other epilepsies. Anticonvulsants should not be started after a concussion to reduce seizure risk. The few studies looking at this question concluded that prophylaxis against seizures is not effective, and most head-injured patients do not develop epilepsy.

EPIDURAL HEMATOMA

The one important danger signal that must be remembered is that peo-ple who are knocked unconscious, regain consciousness, and then lose it again may have an epidural hematoma, a neurosurgical emergency of the highest order (Table 9.2). Epidural hemorrhages are between the dura and the skull and are arterial in origin. They are life-threatening emergencies due to the high pressure. The conscious spell usually lasts only a few minutes so that the PCP would not be involved in the office but could be involved at an athletic event, ski slope, or car accident.

SUBARACHNOID HEMORRHAGE AND SUBDURAL HEMATOMA

Trauma to the head may cause various types of hemorrhages. Traumatic subarachnoid hemorrhage (SAH) is a nonlocalized hemorrhage into the spinal fluid due to multiple capillaries rupturing at the brain's surface. Unlike a subarachnoid hemorrhage from a ruptured aneurysm, a post-traumatic SAH does not often cause problems additional to those caused by the trauma. Subdural hematomas are located outside the brain, between the arachnoid and the dura. These are caused by rupture of veins connecting the dura and the arachnoid and are much more common in the elderly, presumably due to brain atrophy increasing the distance between the dura, which is fixed, and the brain, which can move a little with an impact. These are under low pressure because of the venous origin of the blood.

In the elderly, subdural hematomas (SDHs) may occur with minimal impact. Patients sometimes wonder if there was any impact at all. The symptoms are focal if the hematoma is one-sided, with headache, hemiparesis, or language disorder. The hematomas may resolve, grow, or stay the same size. Because the hematomas have a venous origin and because only a low pressure is required to tamponade the torn vessel, they stop spontaneously. Days or weeks later, the hemorrhaging may resume, without any trauma being remembered. CT scans performed soon after hemorrhage show the white, crescent hematoma. A CT scan, if performed without contrast dye, may show no abnormality during weeks 1–3, because the organizing clot has the same x-ray density as normal brain. Close inspection should reveal some subtle mass effect, with less well-defined sulci on the hematoma side.

Because the elderly are prone to falling, which is the main risk factor for an SDH, the possibility of delayed symptoms must be kept in mind, even when the head trauma was mild. Patients should have a CT scan with and without contrast. An MRI is not necessary. Patients with an SDH should be evaluated by a neurologist or neurosurgeon. If the patient has neurological symptoms or signs (e.g., headache, hemiparesis), then the neurosurgical route should be taken. If the patient is asymptomatic, either consultation is appropriate. Although steroids were once commonly given for this and other post-traumatic brain problems, they are of no value.

CLINICAL PEARLS

- Head trauma causing loss of consciousness followed by regained consciousness and then loss of consciousness is the hallmark of an epidural hematoma, a neurosurgical emergency of the first order.
- Steroids are not useful in treating brain edema due to trauma.
- High-dose steroids are useful for spinal cord injury if started within 8 hours.
- Head trauma is the most common cause of subarachnoid blood seen on CT scan.
- This blood rarely causes the same problems as ruptured aneurysms.
- The term *concussion* has a broad definition that includes mild confusion or amnesia after head trauma, even without loss of consciousness.
- Seizures occurring at the time of the head impact are not a bad prognostic sign either for trauma recovery or for the development of epilepsy.
- Subdural hematomas in the elderly may occur after minimal trauma.
- The AAN recommends that athletes not return to sports activity until 1 week after trauma-induced loss of consciousness.

10

Neuropathies and Myopathies:
Neuromuscular Disease

Disorders of nerve and muscle, aside from pinched nerves and peripheral neuropathies complicating diabetes, are extremely uncommon. In discussing nerve disorders, it is important to distinguish between nerves and roots because the disorders affecting them are generally different. *Root* refers to the nerve fibers that leave the spinal cord. The anterior (motor) portion joins the dorsal or posterior (sensory) portion before exiting the canal. After leaving the canal, the roots in the neck and those in the lumbosacral regions interdigitate to form physically distinct nerve bundles that are each a mixture of roots. In the neck, the roots merge, split, and merge again to ultimately form several nerves including the radial, ulnar, and median nerves, each of which consists of fragments of multiple roots. In the lower back there is only one merge, to form the lumbosacral plexus, consisting of the sciatic, femoral, obturator, and some less clinically important nerves. Roots in the thorax do not merge. They simply travel, as roots, under the appropriate rib. Nerve disorders like mononeuritis multiplex are diseases of individual nerves, such as sciatic, femoral, and ulnar. This is in contrast to disorders of nerve roots (simply called *roots*), such as L3 and C7, that are usually compressive. It should be noted that the motor neuron cell body is located in the spinal cord whereas the sensory neuron resides in a sensory ganglion that is near, but outside, the spinal cord. The sensory neuron sends a dendrite to receive information from the periphery and an axon into the cord to transmit it.

Nerve disorders can be classified in several different ways. Peripheral neuropathies are diffuse conditions affecting the whole body in a relatively symmetric fashion, generally starting distally and gradually ascending from toes to feet to knees before involving the fingers. Peripheral neuropathies can be classified on clinical grounds. Motor neuropathies affect only the nerves innervating muscles. These are rare and may be clinically difficult to distinguish from the lower motor neuron variant of amyotrophic lateral sclerosis. Sensory neuropathies, primarily related to diabetes, cause progressive ascending sensory loss, frequently associated with tingling, altered sensations, or even pain. Some neuropathies involve both motor and sensory modalities and are thus classified as sensory-motor neuropathies. The fourth clinical classification is autonomic. Usually autonomic neuropathies occur in concert with sensory or sensory-motor neuropathies, but may not, and are a common part of diabetes. Peripheral neuropathies are further classified on physiologic and pathologic grounds. Physiologic criteria are based primarily on nerve conduction studies and to a lesser extent on the actual electromyogram (EMG). Disorders of the myelin sheath of the nerve cause a decline in the conduction velocity of the electrical impulse but preserve the amplitude of the motor response in motor neuropathies. Disorders of the axon spare the myelin sheath so that the electrical impulse travels as quickly as it should, but many fibers have no axon so that only a fraction of the impulse is conveyed. Thus, the amplitude of the motor response is diminished. With sensory neuropathies, the same observations are true. This is an oversimplification, however, because prolonged demyelination induces axonal loss, and prolonged axonal loss, especially of larger fibers, leads to the loss of the larger, faster-conducting myelinated fibers, causing a mild slowing of conduction velocity. Thus, the physiologic classification is often unusable as the patient exhibits both slowing and reduced amplitudes, leaving one wondering which is the chicken and which is the egg.

The needle EMG cannot recognize dysfunction of the sensory nerve but is fairly sensitive to axonal loss of the motor neurons. It detects denervation and helps determine if the process is acute (a few months) or chronic (several months or years).

A form of neuropathy that is underrecognized or misidentified as a stroke is an entity called *mononeuropathy* or *mononeuritis* in which isolated nerves are affected. Probably the most common is Bell's palsy, an unexplained, relatively acute peripheral seventh cranial nerve lesion. Isolated nerves, however, can be affected anywhere and are discussed later.

RECOGNIZING NEUROPATHIES AND MYOPATHIES

At their onset peripheral neuropathies are usually asymptomatic. Pain may be early or late, and frequently the patient does not associate neuralgic foot pain with sensory loss. The pain is symmetric and described as a burning or stabbing. The pain is often experienced as feeling like a sunburn and is not problematic until touched. The pain may be worse at night, when even minor stimulation, such as having bed sheets touch the feet, sets off the discomfort. When pain does not bring attention, the earliest symptoms are sensory or motor. The motor symptom is foot weakness or gait dysfunction. Interestingly, many patients notice that they trip or walk abnormally rather than that they have foot drops. Sensory complaints may be indirectly noted: "I drop things," "My hands are clumsy," or "I can't judge how hot the shower is before I get in." Chronic paresthesias, or "pins and needles," are often perceived as a circulation problem. Autonomic dysfunction is manifest primarily in terms of orthostatic lightheadedness or dizziness (see Chapter 4), incontinence, or sexual dysfunction, particularly erectile dysfunction in men.

Most peripheral neuropathies cause symmetric distal painless numbness or weakness. The examination should take this into account by focusing on the toes and the feet. Toe strength may be reduced and intrinsic foot muscles may atrophy and reveal fasciculations, which are random contractions of single motor units that look like slight ripples under the skin. Fasciculations do not induce limb movements. They are sometimes induced by tapping a muscle but their appearance is unpredictable. Tone in peripheral nerve disorders is always normal or reduced. Contractions such as claw hand or tight tendons rarely develop from nerve disorders. Toe strength is tested in extension and flexion. Then the five muscles moving the foot are tested (anterior tibialis for dorsiflexion, posterior tibialis for inversion, gastrocnemius and soleus for plantar flexion, and peronei muscles for eversion). The ankle jerk is checked and is often absent in both sensorimotor and sensory neuropathies. Sensation is tested as described in Appendix 1, but with greater diligence. Light touch, temperature, and position sense are checked. Vibration is probably the most sensitive indicator of sensation but is so often impaired in the otherwise normal elderly that it must be severely impaired in an elderly patient before I attach significance to it. Position sense testing is particularly useful in assessing gait abnormalities (Table 10.1).

It is difficult to quantify sensory impairment. There are now devices that have electrically controlled vibratory simulators that can be used to reliably determine the degree of impairment. What is probably more important, however, is how proximal the deficit is. Therefore, I recommend marching a pin from foot up to thigh to determine the level, a test that can then be used in follow-up for determining progression. Because few neuropathies are treatable, this is something of an academic exercise, but it may allow for interpretation of patient deficits and their relationship to the neuropathy. It is important to realize that simply recognizing sharp from dull is not an adequate test of sensory function. A pain may be perceived as sharper proximally than distally but still may be sharp in the toe. One also must note that a dysesthetic response may be painful so that a pinprick may be more painful distally, yet temperature sensation, which is carried over the same fibers, may be reduced. This is due to the sensory abnormality in which one stimulus is misperceived. That is, the nerve carries an impaired message to the spinal cord, transforming *sharp* to *pain*, not *sharp* to *extra*

Table 10.1. Peripheral neuropathy vs. muscle disease

	Peripheral neuropathy	*Muscle disease*
Atrophy	Yes	No
Fasciculations	Common	Rare
Tendon reflexes	Absent	Normal or decreased
Sensory loss	Often	Never
Autonomic dysfunction	Occasional	Never
Dysphagia	Rare	Occasional
Gait abnormalities	Wide based; high stepping	Waddling; hyperlordosis
Creatine phosphokinase elevation	Occasional	Usual
Trophic changes*	Common	Never

*Trophic changes are skeletal and joint changes due to chronic injury or abnormal stress and include Charcot joints, hammer toes, and high arches.

sharp or *painfully sharp*. Localization of the stimulation is typically reduced in this setting.

Clinical evaluation of autonomic function is limited. Blood pressure measurements are taken with the patient seated and standing at 1, 2, and 3 minutes. A 15-point systolic drop or greater is considered significant. There are several reasons for orthostatic hypotension, however, and only a few of them are neurologic. Dehydration and antihypertensive drugs are the most common causes. An autonomic neuropathy should cause, in addition to the drop in blood pressure, no compensatory increase in heart rate, which occurs with the previously named causes of orthostatic hypotension except when beta-blocking drugs are used. Rectal tone may or may not be impaired with an autonomic neuropathy. The bulbocavernosus reflex, in which the anus contracts when the glans penis is squeezed, may be impaired. Dry skin may be a sign of autonomic dysfunction, as may pupillary abnormalities and failure to sweat appropriately.

COMPRESSIVE NEUROPATHIES

Pinched nerves are the most common peripheral nerve symptoms and are usually responsive to treatment. Disk herniations and arthritic bone growth press on nerves in the spinal canal. This occurs in the lumbosacral spine and neck and very rarely in the thorax. This topic is discussed in Chapter 3, because the syndrome of nerve compression in the spine is almost always associated with pain. The other common compressive neuropathies are median nerve entrapment in the wrist, causing carpal tunnel syndrome and cubital (elbow) entrapment of the ulnar nerve.

Carpal Tunnel Syndrome and Ulnar Entrapment

Carpal tunnel syndrome (CTS) is a common disorder that has been increasingly recognized in recent years as a workplace injury due to repetitive movements involving wrist flexion. Although there are predisposing conditions for CTS such as diabetes, arthritis of all types, and hypothyroidism, most CTS patients have no medical predisposing risk factors, and many have no identifiable repetitive motion risk factors. The usual symptoms are tingling and numbness in the hand, described as feeling like "bad circulation." The symptoms commonly awaken the patient at night. The patient often then flicks the hand (the "wrist flick sign") to "get the circulation going." Symptoms can also occur during the day while the patient drives or holds a newspaper. Occasional patients can localize the numbness to the median nerve distribution (the palmar surface of the palm and fingers from the thumb to half of the ring finger) but most perceive the whole hand as being involved. The hand may also ache. Although the muscle in the thenar eminence (the abductor pollicis brevis) may be atrophied, the patient rarely perceives weakness because there are several muscles that move the thumb. Pain in the wrist, often radiating up the arm, is common. The examination is often normal, but sensory changes in the median distribution and the size of the abductor pollicis brevis should be checked.

The ulnar nerve, which travels around the elbow, is what causes the pain when one hits his or her "funny bone." This nerve travels in the cubital groove and may stretch with prolonged elbow flexion or get compressed in the forearm. Patients usually have elbow pain radiating into the hand or into the upper arm and numbness in the medial (ulnar) aspect of the hand, splitting the ring finger. Weakness in the interosseous muscles, which separate the fingers, is part of the syndrome but less common.

Both CTS and ulnar entrapment may be very symptomatic, with little or nothing abnormal on examination. Tinel's sign (tingling and pain on tapping the point of compression) is not a reliable sign. The diagnosis of both these syndromes rests on the EMG. Nerve conduction studies show a delay in the conduction speed across the point of compression on both motor and sensory studies. The needle EMG is used primarily for excluding radiculopathies or double crush syndromes, in which there is both a proximal nerve lesion plus the distal entrapment. CTS is frequently bilateral even when only one side is symptomatic.

Management

Nerve entrapment can be approached conservatively at first. CTS can be managed with wrist splints and reduction of repetitive flexing tasks. Should these fail, some specialists use steroid injections while others recommend surgical release. Surgery cures the symptoms in the vast majority of patients. Ulnar entrapment can be approached with a towel wrapped around the elbow at night to prevent elbow flexing with nerve stretching. Should this fail and if no predisposing factor is found, such as resting the upper forearm on a hard edge, then surgery is recommended. This is more complicated than CTS repair because the nerve is moved from behind to the front of the elbow.

Mononeuropathy and Mononeuritis Multiplex

There are two important reasons for recognizing a mononeuritis multiplex. One is that it is usually a more benign syndrome than a stroke, with which it is usually confused. The second is that it may mimic a tumor compressing a nerve. In a mononeuritis multiplex, one or more nerves suddenly become dysfunctional. This is usually painless but, as in the case of brachial neuralgia, may be quite painful. Presumably, any nerve may be affected, but certain ones are more commonly affected. Bell's palsy, or idiopathic facial nerve palsy, is the most common. Patients complain of pain behind the ear and numbness on the cheek but are found on examination to have isolated weakness of the muscles of facial expression on one side, with widened palpebral fissure, decreased nasolabial fold, and diminished ability to raise the eyebrow (the distinguishing feature from an upper motor neuron facial weakness). Despite the symptom of numbness, none is found on examination. Other isolated cranial neuropathies are rare aside from a third nerve palsy associated with diabetes. The so-called *diabetic third* (nerve palsy) is phenomenologically unusual in that all third nerve functions are impaired except for the pupil. It is therefore a pupil-sparing third nerve palsy. The eyelid is closed, and when the lid is opened the eye is externally deviated and cannot move up, down, or medially, but the pupil is intact. Retro-orbital pain is common. Unfortunately, occasional posterior communicating aneurysms can cause the same syndrome although they usually involve the pupil, causing a clinical conundrum of what tests to perform in this case. My own recommendations are to obtain a conventional arteriogram if the patient does not have diabetes, and a noninvasive magnetic resonance angiogram if the patient is diabetic.

Femoral neuropathies are common diabetic complications but may occur without diabetes, raising the question of a vasculitis. This is usually a painless syndrome of weakness in the femoral distribution—namely, hip flexion and lower leg extension—with loss of the knee jerk and possible anterior thigh sensory loss. The hip adductors and abductors should be strong. The clinical distinction between a femoral nerve lesion and an L3 or L4 radiculopathy may be impossible to make, necessitating an EMG. The EMG can determine if paraspinal muscles are denervated, indicating a root abnormality, or if L3 or L4 innervated muscles outside a femoral nerve distribution are involved subclinically.

Sciatic nerve mononeuritis is less common than femoral and far less common than radiculopathies of L4 or L5, causing sciatic symptoms. The major other mononeuritis multiplex syndromes are lumbosacral plexus and brachial plexus syndromes. The latter is a painful shoulder syndrome that does not improve with position changes and may be exacerbated by some arm movements. The distribution of the weakness, wasting, and sensory loss is a function of which parts of the plexus are involved. The importance of localizing the process to the plexus, which is done by demonstrating that the pattern of denervation is not in a root distribution and fits better with a nerve, cord, or trunk lesion, is that the evaluation then focuses on excluding an apical lung tumor or infiltrating carcinoma as the etiology. The lumbosacral plexus is another site where a similar, although usually painless, mononeuritis occurs.

A relatively common, benign, but interesting, mononeuritis is meralgia paresthetica, a sensory syndrome of the lateral cutaneous nerve of the thigh. The clinical syndrome is an aching numbness with dysesthesias in an elliptical distribution on the lateral thigh. There is no motor component or reflex change. The numbness is bothersome and may be permanent. It had been associated primarily with obese women who wore tight fitting corsets until fashions changed. It is now associated with substantial weight loss or is idiopathic and occurs in both men and women. Sigmund Freud suffered from this condition.

Multiple mononeuropathies in the nondiabetic patient deserve expedited work-up, meaning prompt referral to a neurologist to exclude vasculitis or other potentially severe illness.

The pathophysiology of mononeuritis multiplex is postulated to be nerve infarct, but this has not been proved. Most patients with mononeuritis syndromes recover, but not all.

POLYNEUROPATHIES

There are a large number of systemic disorders associated with neuropathies. Diabetes is by far the most common. Typically, it causes a sensory neuropathy that is evident on evaluation. Autonomic dysfunction can be elicited by a history of erectile dysfunction in men or by measuring orthostatic blood pressure. Nutritional disorders may cause neuropathies, with vitamin B_{12} and pyridoxine the best described. Alcoholics develop neuropathy that is most likely due to nutritional deficiency rather than alcohol toxicity. Certain drugs commonly cause neuropathy. The anticancer drugs vincristine and cisplatin always cause this unwanted adverse effect. Isoniazid, given for tuberculosis, frequently causes a sensory neuropathy within a few weeks of drug initiation due to interference with pyridoxine and is reversed by pyridoxine supplementation. Phenytoin (Dilantin) occasionally causes an asymptomatic neuropathy. Many chemicals are toxic to the nervous system, with lead and organic solvents being the most common. Lead causes a motor neuropathy that affects the hands more often than the legs and may mimic motor neuron disease. In adults it does not usually cause an encephalopathy. Other heavy-metal salts may also induce neuropathies but are not often seen. Metabolic disorders, particularly uremia, cause neuropathies. Probably all patients with chronic renal failure have sensory or sensory motor neuropathies. Hypothyroidism, systemic amyloidosis, and porphyria are rare causes of neuropathy and do not generally have neuropathy as the presenting feature. A variety of systemic illnesses may have neuropathies as their initial symptom, however, including collagen vascular diseases, such as lupus or polyarteritis nodosa; paraneoplastic syndromes with known or occult primaries; sarcoidosis; and paraproteinemias. Infections other than Lyme disease are rare causes of neuropathy. Lyme disease may induce neuropathy in 10–15% of cases. Diphtheria and leprosy are exceedingly uncommon in the Western world these days. Human immunodeficiency virus (HIV) as well as its drug therapies may cause neuropathies. A spectrum of inherited disorders with the patterns of autosomal dominant, recessive, X-linked, or mitochondrial (maternal) inheritance are also associated with neuropathies. Because these may be X-linked or recessive there may be no family history. In the intensive care unit setting, an entity called *critical illness polyneuropathy* may complicate the picture of the critically ill, often septic patient who had been intubated for several days. Frequently, the patient was sedated intermittently. On attempting to wean the patient, diffuse weakness becomes apparent due to a sensorimotor neuropathy. Finally, elderly people often have a mild sensory neuropathy that is considered normal.

GUILLAIN-BARRÉ SYNDROME

Most neuropathies are very slowly progressive and insidious in onset. Guillain-Barré syndrome (GBS) is one of the few neuropathies that develops rapidly. Others are toxin and angiitis-induced neuropathies, which are exceedingly rare. GBS is the only relatively acute neuropathy common enough to consider. GBS is usually an ascending polyneuropathy. It starts in the feet and then progresses upward, affecting the hands once it ascends above the knees. It primarily affects people in the sixth through eighth decades, but it may affect children. Patients develop ascending weakness, usually accompanied by sensory symptoms and signs; loss of deep tendon reflexes; and elevated protein in the spinal fluid. About 60% have a preceding viral upper respiratory or gastrointestinal syndrome. Usually the syndrome progresses over days to weeks and therefore usually presents as an outpatient disorder; however, fulminant cases evolving over hours may occur. The severity of the disorder varies enormously. Patients with severe cases become respirator dependent, whereas patients with milder cases never require hospitalization. All cases of presumed GBS should be referred to a neurologist. If there is a question about the rate of progression, the patient should be hospitalized and pulmonary function tests need to be monitored. GBS severe enough to prevent walking has been shown to improve more readily with plasmapheresis or intravenous immunoglobin than without any intervention. These are expensive therapies that should only be employed by experts. Generally, GBS reaches its nadir by week 4 and then slowly improves, leaving little residue when mild but prominent weakness when the patient has been severely impaired.

ASSESSING A NEUROPATHY

Mild diabetic neuropathies and mild sensory decline in the elderly require no further evaluation. Other cases should generally be referred to a neurologist for evaluation. The obvious possible etiologies, however, should be considered first. Diabetes may in fact present with the neuropathy. With erectile dysfunction such a common complication, men occasionally present with this symptom rather than weight loss, polydipsia, or polyuria. Systemic distal pain due to the neuropathy may be the presenting feature in diabetes, and diabetic amyotrophy frequently occurs before diabetes has been diagnosed.

An EMG is useful primarily for determining the extent of motor involvement. The sensory component of testing usually does little more than confirm the existence of the neuropathy. By the time the exam reveals the typical stocking distal loss, the sensory nerve action potentials are usually absent in the feet. The nerve conduction study may reveal abnormalities in the hand or arm that are not clinically apparent. The motor nerve conduction studies may reveal whether the neurologic process is demyelinating or axonal, or whether the process is uniform or patchy, each of which may point to a diagnosis. The needle EMG picks up evidence of denervation that tells how widespread the process is and how chronic or acute.

Routine blood tests should include vitamin B_{12} and folate levels, thyroid functions (to exclude hypothyroidism), fasting blood sugar, erythrocyte sedimentation rate, antinuclear antibody as screening tests for vasculitis and occult cancer, and serum protein electrophoresis and serum immunoelectrophoresis for paraproteinemias. Nonroutine blood tests may include antinerve antibodies: the anti–myelin-associated glycoprotein should be considered in middle-aged to older adults with sensorimotor neuropathy; the anti-GM_1 (ganglioside component of myelin) should be considered in motor neuropathies. Genetic tests, which are becoming increasingly available in commercial laboratories, may be indicated in rare cases. These expensive and sophisticated tests should be reserved for a neurologist.

Table 10.2. Signs and symptoms of peripheral nerve disorders

Type of Involvement	Signs	Symptoms
Sensory	Decreased sensation, distal > proximal	Numbness; tingling, burning
		Parasthesias
	Clumsiness and ataxia	Abnormal gait; clumsiness
	Loss of tendon reflexes	
	Loss of nociceptive responses (e.g., Babinski)	
	Trophic changes	
Autonomic	Orthostatic hypotension without heart rate compensation	Fainting
		Constipation, diarrhea, bloating
	Sweating abnormalities	Hyper- or hypotension
	Pupil abnormalities	
Motor	Atrophy, fasciculations	Impotence; incontinence
	Hypotonia	Weakness; cramps
	Scoliosis	Weight loss

Occasionally a lumbar puncture may be required. Many neuropathies are associated with elevated cerebrospinal fluid protein, but none are associated with pleocytosis unless the neuropathy is of a systemic illness such as vasculitis. GBS produces very high protein levels without a pleocytosis.

Nerve biopsies are particularly useful in diagnosing inflammatory neuropathies. Because there may be an effective treatment, a definitive diagnosis is of more than academic interest. However, there are a limited number of nerves to biopsy, and the most commonly studied—the sural, which is in the ankle and foot—is frequently so severely affected that its histology is nondiagnostic. A neurologist with special interest in nerve disorders should be involved in this decision.

Other considerations depend on the clinical situation (Table 10.2). A very large number of disorders are associated with neuropathies, and most are excluded in the history. Porphyria, for example, is rare and is associated with abdominal pain and psychosis. Toxins are rare except in a few occupations. Lyme disease, on the other hand, is common in certain regions and frequently has peripheral neuropathy associated with it. HIV and its drug treatments also may be associated with neuropathies. Hence, the testing performed depends on the clinical setting. Many neuropathies remain undiagnosed even after every diagnostic study, including nerve biopsy, has been obtained. Failure to make a diagnosis even at an aggressive, university-based neuromuscular disease service is quite common.

TREATMENT

Treatment for neuropathies is dissatisfying. Treating an underlying systemic disease halts the progression and sometimes reverses it, but rarely to normal. Controlling diabetes makes little clinical difference in diabetic neuropathy. Treatment of monoclonal gammopathies and cancers may or may not improve the neuropathy, whereas nutritional improvement in deficiency states and discontinuation of an offending drug or toxin stops progression and possibly leads to improvement. Common sense suggestions are more important. Some suggestions are proper care of toes to guard against painless infections, physical therapy assessments for ankle braces, and home safety evaluations. Symptomatic therapy for neuropathic pain syndromes, usually with carbamazepine, tricyclic antidepressants, capsaicin, or gabapentin, may be extremely gratifying.

MYOPATHIES

Muscle disorders are rare. Even excluding the diabetic neuropathies, muscle disorders are rarer than neuropathies. Patients typically complain of painless weakness. Early in the course, this weakness is evident to the patient but not to the examining physician. Demanding tasks such as climbing onto a chair may be well performed. The patient complaining of weakness often describes easy fatigability, a symptom seen in so many systemic, neurologic, and psychiatric disorders that it may be useless or even misleading in diagnosis. When weakness becomes evident it is usually proximal. One unusual feature of myopathies is that neck flexors are affected early and much more than neck extensors. Muscle bulk usually is unchanged. Muscle tone is unchanged. Deep tendon reflexes are normal or mildly reduced. Cramps are common in muscle disorders but are common enough in neuropathic disorders that they are not diagnostic features. Myotonia, however, which is a painless tonic contraction of a muscle, or, more accurately, the inability to relax a muscle contracted voluntarily, is a sign of muscle disease. Muscle pain, aside from that associated with cramps, is distinctly unusual in muscle disorders. It is a common misperception that polymyositis, because it is an inflammatory disorder, must be painful, but it is not. Some muscle disorders affect the extraocular muscles, causing a group of disorders called progressive external ophthalmoplegias, which are rare. Their characteristic feature is bilateral ptosis and, of course, impaired eye movement.

Muscle diseases are either acquired or the result of inborn errors of metabolism. The inherited disorders are myopathies and have variable ages of onset. Because they are due to single gene abnormalities, their inheritance pattern may be autosomal dominant, autosomal recessive, X-linked recessive, or mitochondrial (maternally inherited only). Because of the possibility of adult-onset signs and symptoms and the possibly negative family history, these seemingly sporadic cases may be difficult to diagnose. Some of the disorders involve more than skeletal muscles. Early cataracts, hypogonadism, mild retardation, eye movement weakness, and cardiac problems all may complicate the picture and generally point to a systemic biochemical and thus inherited disorder. The acquired disorders are, although still rare, more likely to be encountered by the average primary care physician. They are inflammatory, toxin- or drug-induced, and endocrine associated.

Inflammatory Myopathies

Inflammatory myopathies include polymyositis, dermatomyositis, sarcoidosis, and some toxic and inherited disorders. They are considered inflammatory based on the histologic finding of lymphocytic infiltration of muscle. Polymyositis and dermatomyositis, although still rare, are the only ones worth considering here. It is estimated that there are only 5–10 new cases of all inflammatory myopathies per million people per year. This translates to fewer than 10 new cases per year in my home state of Rhode Island. Polymyositis and dermatomyositis have similar clinical features, with peak incidence in middle age, but dermatomyositis also affects children and is associated with a rash. Both have an insidious onset over weeks to months. There is usually no pain. Weakness affects proximal muscles more than distal muscles, including neck flexors. Swallowing problems occur in almost half the patients. A lung or the heart may become involved. Dermatomyositis is associated with increased risk of malignancy, but polymyositis is not. Cancer is present or occurs in 25% of dermatomyositis patients. The major feature distinguishing polymyositis from dermatomyositis is the rash. The rash may precede or accompany the muscle manifestations of dermatomyositis. The heliotrope rash is a purple discoloration around the eyes, particularly the upper lids, often associated with periorbital edema. Other skin manifestations include reddish-purple papules over bony prominences, particularly over the knuckles, but also over the elbows, knees, and ankles. Periungual telangiectasia and a photosensitive face and chest rash may also occur. Heart involvement occurs in half the patients with either disorder, causing rhythm problems or congestive heart failure.

Diagnosis

Diagnosis of inflammatory myopathy is based on muscle biopsy. The creatine phosphokinase (CPK) should be elevated. The EMG is helpful, showing widespread fibrillations (typical of acute neuropathy or inflammatory myopathy) and myopathic potentials, but the biopsy is required for a firm diagnosis and should be required before initiating therapy.

A variety of serologic test results may be abnormal in polymyositis and dermatomyositis, particularly in the 25% of patients who have an associated collagen vascular disease or malignancy. In some patients, the titers of these tests parallel the activity of cancer or the collagen vascular disease.

The need for an occult malignancy evaluation is still under debate. Most authorities suggest a screen for malignancy with a physical examination, including rectal and pelvic examinations and laboratory studies including mammogram, chest x-ray, prostate-specific antigen, stool for occult blood, urinalysis, and complete blood count.

Treatment

Therapy is aimed at the presumed immune origin of the disease. Because the natural history of these disorders is unknown, the benefits of treatment are unclear. In mild, relatively asymptomatic disease, possibly picked up by a screening CPK abnormality, the patient may be followed expectantly. In most cases prednisone is used, with azathioprine as backup if steroids produce no response. Chronic steroid use leads to its own well-known problems, including steroid myopathy. Steroid myopathy is distinguished from polymyositis by increased weakness without a CPK elevation and without the inflammatory EMG changes. There are nonspecific features, however, and the final diagnosis may rest on the clinical course after tapering or discontinuing the steroids.

Inclusion body myositis is another inflammatory myopathy that has a distinctive pathology and, although uncommon, is important to recognize because of its refractoriness to steroid therapy.

Other Myopathies

Other myopathies are even less common than the inflammatory ones and are mentioned only for completeness. Steroid-induced myopathy is associated with other steroid stigmata such as a buffalo hump, central obesity, and osteoporosis, and patients must have been on a glucocorticoid. Hypothyroidism, hyperthyroidism, hyperparathyroidism, and growth hormone excess are endocrine myopathies. A variety of drugs, including azidothymidine, cyclosporine, ethanol, D-penicillamine, and hypervitaminosis E, may cause myopathy. A large number of inborn errors of metabolism may cause isolated muscle disease or systemic disorders with muscle involvement. These may be diagnosed by sophisticated metabolic studies in some cases or by muscle biopsy. In the future, many cases will be diagnosed by gene testing.

CLINICAL PEARLS

- Myopathies usually cause proximal weakness.
- Neuropathies usually cause distal weakness.
- A pupil-sparing third nerve palsy is most likely due to diabetes (ptosis, eye deviated laterally but normal pupil).
- The diagnosis of CTS does not mandate an evaluation for diabetes, thyroid disease, or other systemic disorders.
- Myopathies frequently cause neck flexor weakness early in their course.
- Inflammatory myopathies are not usually painful.
- Myopathies may or may not reduce deep tendon reflexes. Neuropathies always do.
- Neither neuropathies nor myopathies cause positive Babinski reflexes or increased deep tendon reflexes.
- Myopathies do not affect sensation.
- Neuropathies may cause atrophy and fasciculations. Myopathies do not cause fasciculations and cause wasting only after a long duration.

11

Famous Diseases

This chapter reviews several neurologic disorders that are either encountered or discussed frequently. I have specifically not attempted to integrate these diseases (except Alzheimer's disease) into other chapters, although relevant aspects of these diseases may be discussed elsewhere. For example, Parkinson's disease and normal pressure hydrocephalus are discussed in Chapter 5 on gait disorders. I believe that primary care physicians (PCPs) often worry about not having encountered many well-known disorders and wonder if they are missing diagnoses, unaware that many are so rare that neurologists often do not see them either. Nevertheless, these disorders are well-known and recognizable and are sometimes treatable. Even when the disorder is not treatable, patients are usually reassured that they have an identifiable illness. Having a name to attach to their syndrome is a relief to most patients. It allows the patient to access further information and patient support on the Internet and elsewhere. Patients suspected of having these disorders should always be referred for a formal neurologic assessment and treatment plan.

MYASTHENIA GRAVIS

Myasthenia gravis (MG) is a rare disease that has a prevalence of 40–80 per million and an uncertain incidence, estimated at 1–3 per million to 2–10 per 100,000. This puts it in the ballpark of Jacob-Creutzfeldt disease in terms of incidence. Since most myasthenics survive for decades, the prevalence is considerably higher. Although patients complain of varying degrees of weakness and fatigue, the most common symptoms are related to the eyes, with half of patients presenting with

Table 11.1. Myasthenia gravis

Very rare
Varying degrees of ptosis and diplopia
Varying degree of limb weakness
Fatigue
Progressive weakness with effort

impaired eye movement (diplopia) or eyelid droop (ptosis). Virtually all patients have eye involvement at some point. Patients may be confused by the intermittency of the problem, perhaps seeing an optometrist or ophthalmologist during a period when nothing is wrong. Muscles of the throat are next most commonly affected, causing a nasal voice or dysphagia, which is particularly true for thin liquids. This may produce nasal regurgitation of water (Table 11.1).

MG falls into two clinical syndromes: a form that is restricted only to the eyes and the more common generalized form that involves the eyes plus skeletal musculature. The disease has clearly been shown to be an autoimmune disorder due to an antibody directed against skeletal muscle acetylcholine receptors. On electron microscopy the receptor is seen to be in a deteriorated state.

Generalized MG usually affects young to middle-aged adults, but children and older people may also be affected. In addition to eye and throat involvement, striated skeletal muscle is affected. This causes a variable amount of weakness in different muscle groups that changes over time. The weakness is usually more proximal than distal so that symptoms include difficulty climbing stairs, getting out of a chair, and lifting heavy objects. Smooth muscle and cardiac muscle are completely spared so that bladder and bowel dysfunction do not occur. Heart function is normal as well. An important diagnostic point is the sparing of the smooth muscles of the iris, thus maintaining normal pupil function in the face of ptosis and eye movement weakness, implying that the problem is not due to third cranial nerve (oculomotor) dysfunction. Another important diagnostic clue is the easy fatigability that is distinct from usual complaints of fatigue in that repeated exercise produces true weakness, not simply a generalized weak feeling.

MG is diagnosed with a variety of tests. The standard edrophonium test, in which a small intravenous dose of this cholinesterase inhibitor (hence, a cholinergic activator) transiently increases strength, should be performed by an experienced person. The PCP who suspects MG should send serum for an acetylcholine receptor antibody titer and acquire a chest computed tomography (CT) scan and thyroid function tests because there is an association between thyroid disease and MG. The chest CT is required for two reasons. There is a risk of thymoma with MG, and many patients are treated with thymectomies for generalized MG for immune reasons, even if no thymoma is seen. The neurologist usually checks the muscle response to repetitive electrical shocks during the electromyogram (EMG), because repeated shocks deplete the muscle endplate of acetylcholine. The single-fiber EMG is probably the most sensitive laboratory test for MG.

Treatment should be rendered by someone experienced because MG patients can get very sick very quickly and face emergencies due to pulmonary compromise. Choosing when to change steroid doses, institute plasmapheresis or intravenous immunoglobulin, hospitalize the patient, and so forth is often extremely difficult and requires an experienced neurologist.

A clinically similar but actually "opposite" syndrome is the Lambert-Eaton myasthenic syndrome, in which patients develop MG symptoms although the disorder usually spares the eyes. These patients actually become stronger with repetitive contractions, a mirror image of MG, in which strength declines. This rare syndrome, initially noted as a paraneoplastic syndrome, actually is more common without an associated malignancy. It is commonly associated with other autoimmune problems such as thyroiditis, vitiligo, pernicious anemia, and rheumatoid arthritis.

Table 11.2.   Parkinson's disease

Common, particularly in the elderly
Patients are slow and look depressed
Gait slows, arm swing is reduced
Posture is stooped
Tremor at rest in most patients, but not all
Should be considered in patients older than 50 with gait, slowness,
    clumsiness, or fatigue symptoms

PARKINSON'S DISEASE

Parkinson's disease (PD) is a common disorder affecting about 1%
of the white American population over the age of 60. It affects men
preferentially, at a ratio of about 1.5 to 1.0, and appears to be less
common in African Americans and Africans. Asian populations are
affected about equally to Europeans and white Americans. With this
high a prevalence, every physician who sees adult patients sees
patients with PD (Table 11.2).

The median age at onset is 60, and about 5% of patients develop
the illness before the age of 40 (young-onset PD). Although there is
more known about this neurodegenerative disease than any other,
there is precious little yet known. The cause is unknown. For a long
time, a viral or slow virus etiology was suspected, and a link to the
great Spanish influenza epidemic at the end of World War I was proposed, but this concept has been abandoned. There is a very rare form
of PD that is inherited as an autosomal dominant trait, and one gene
has been identified. The current theory of etiology in noninherited PD
is that the cause lies in a problem with oxidative phosphorylation. This,
however, remains a hypothesis. Therapy is aimed at symptoms, not at
arresting progression. PD is always progressive, but the variability of
progression is enormous, ranging from patients who are wheelchair-
bound in 5 years to those only mildly affected after 20 years.

PD is a brain disorder in which a very restricted region of the
brain is affected. The predominant cell type affected produces the
neurotransmitter dopamine, resulting in a dopamine deficiency state.

Drugs that block dopamine receptors, such as antipsychotics, or deplete dopamine, such as the antihypertensive drug reserpine, produce clinical states that look exactly like PD but are not progressive and always reverse on drug discontinuation.

PD usually is asymmetric, starting on one side and then remaining more severe on the first affected side. Although most people think of PD as being primarily a tremor disorder, tremor does not occur in all patients. About 80% of PD patients do have tremor; thus, 20% do not. Tremor is usually more a cosmetic than a functional problem, but it does bring the patient to medical attention. Tremor occurs at rest and resolves with movement. It affects fingers, hands, and the chin, in that order of frequency. It does not involve the head. The other cardinal features of PD are hypokinesia (akinesia, meaning absence of movement, and bradykinesia, meaning slowness of movement), rigidity (not always with cog-wheeling), posture, and balance problems. PD patients look depressed or angry, even when they are not. The voice usually loses volume and speech may become stuttered. PD is the most common cause of adult-acquired stuttering. Handwriting deteriorates due to tremor, poor coordination, and micrographia. Balance and posture problems are described in Chapter 5.

About half of PD patients develop depression and about one-third become demented. Although depression occurs at all stages of the disease, dementia tends to occur in advanced disease, particularly in the elderly. The depression responds to antidepressants just as it does in age-matched non-PD patients.

PD is always progressive, but the variation in course is impressive. In general, if signs and symptoms begin slowly, they tend to remain slow in their progression throughout the course. Longevity is only mildly diminished in general, and death occurs either from unrelated diseases or secondary conditions, particularly pneumonia, or from complications of hip fracture.

Treatment of PD is symptomatic. There are theoretical concerns that, although L-dopa is the single most effective treatment, it may be harmful in the long run. As a result of this concern, most (but not all) PD specialists shy away from using L-dopa when there is little functional impairment, especially in young patients, reserving its use for patients with significant disability. For older patients, concern over long-term complications related to L-dopa are inappropriate, allowing earlier use of the drug. At some point, usually within 1 year of diagnosis, all patients require L-dopa or one of the dopamine agonists. Over time most patients require multiple PD drugs.

It is often thought that L-dopa is only useful for 3–5 years. This is incorrect and represents a misunderstanding of the fact that by 3–5 years, half the patients taking L-dopa have some drug-related complications. In most cases, these are mild. Only in very advanced disease does L-dopa stop working. This is due to the absence of any nigral cells left to take up the L-dopa that is inactive and convert it to dopamine. Although selegiline was originally thought to slow disease progression, this was not borne out by longer-term studies. Thus, therapy centers around treating symptoms, which usually means a dopamine agonist (bromocriptine, pergolide, pramipexole, or ropinerole) or L-dopa. Anticholinergics are often used for treating tremor but are not useful for the other aspects of PD that are usually more important. In addition, anticholinergics cause dry mouth, constipation, frequently urinary retention, blurred vision, and memory impairment.

Daily walking is very important, as is maintenance of an active lifestyle. PD patients tend to become increasingly withdrawn, and, if they are not forced to socialize, often become reclusive.

AMYOTROPHIC LATERAL SCLEROSIS

Amyotrophic lateral sclerosis (ALS, also known as Lou Gehrig's disease) is the single most common variant of the motor neuron diseases (MNDs), and although the terms are often used synonymously, MND is clearly more than a single disease. MND refers to four distinct syndromes: spinal muscular atrophy, ALS, progressive muscular atrophy (PMA), and progressive lateral sclerosis. As the name suggests, MND is a set of disorders involving motor neurons. Clinically, one sees progressive, painless loss of strength and atrophy resulting from the loss of motor neurons in the spinal cord or the brain. ALS is

Table 11.3.   Amyotrophic lateral sclerosis

Rare; affects men and women
Usually occurs in middle age
Painless, progressive weakness and atrophy
Affects muscles above and below the neck

the clinical syndrome associated with the degeneration of both cortical motor neurons and lower motor neurons. The upper, or cortical,
motor neuron loss leads to weakness with increased reflexes and
positive Babinski reflexes, whereas the degeneration of brain stem
motor nuclei and motor neurons in the anterior portion of the spinal
cord leads to weakness with atrophy, fasciculations, and the loss of
reflexes. The combined picture of atrophy, weakness, fasciculations,
and hyperflexia is highly suggestive of ALS. PMA is the other major
variant of MND in adults and is a primarily lower motor neuron
form of the disease. The famous physicist Stephen Hawking has this
variant, as did Jacob Javits, the former senator from New York.
While the weakness is the same as in ALS, reflexes are diminished,
the Babinski reflexes are not present, and fasciculations are widespread. ALS, which kills within 1–3 years, is a more rapidly progressive disorder than PMA, which occasionally progresses over many
years (Table 11.3).

ALS has an incidence of about 1.5 per 100,000 per year throughout the world, affecting men more than women, at a ratio of about
1.5 to 1.0. It generally affects the middle-aged population and carries
a life expectancy of less than 3 years. About 10% of cases are inherited as an autosomal dominant disorder, so that 90% of cases are
sporadic without apparent genetic influence. The gene for familial
ALS has been identified and is being actively studied for the insights
it might shed on the more common sporadic form.

ALS patients usually begin their disease with focal weakness, typically in the hands before the weakness spreads proximally. Sometimes it begins in the feet or in the pharynx. Initially there may be a
significant degree of asymmetry—for example, a single foot drop—

causing diagnostic confusion, but over time the weakness spreads contralaterally and proximally. The upper motor neuron degeneration causes reflex changes but little in the way of symptoms. Sensation is spared, although patients may have minor sensory symptoms. Eye muscles, both intrinsic (pupils) and extrinsic (extraocular movements), are spared. Occasionally bladder urgency or incontinence may occur, but this is not the rule, and its occurrence should cause questions about the diagnosis (see the section on differential diagnosis below). The disease is always progressive and tends to progress in a linear fashion over time. The bulbar variant, which affects structures (the throat and tongue) innervated by nuclei in the bulb or medulla, is the most rapidly progressive, probably due to the earlier development of aspiration.

The diagnosis of ALS is clinical. The differential diagnostic list is limited. The major concern is distinguishing ALS from cervical spondylosis (see Chapter 3), which causes a clinical myelopathy with weakness, wasting, and fasciculations in the arms and spasticity of the legs. Often, patients with cervical spine disease also have lumbar stenosis, causing wasting or fasciculations in the legs. Atrophy and fasciculations in the tongue or facial weakness, however, clearly imply a process occurring above the spinal cord. Because the cranial nerves cannot be compressed in the neck, the diagnosis becomes unavoidable. Peripheral neuropathies occurring in patients with spasticity may also mimic ALS.

Any patient with suspected ALS should be referred to a neurologist promptly to make a definitive diagnosis. The essence of the diagnosis is the EMG showing widespread denervation in arms, legs, and, most important, the tongue. Treatment is mainly supportive, although one medication, riluzole, has been shown to minimally slow disease progression. Cognitive function and eye movements remain intact throughout the disease. Autonomic functions also remain intact, but inability to move leads to urinary incontinence. Abdominal weakness and lack of ambulation lead to constipation.

Spinal muscular atrophy is the pure lower motor neuron form of MND occurring in children and represents a group of diseases. The most common form, which is inherited as an autosomal recessive trait, occurs in infancy and childhood and bears the eponymic names of Werdnig-Hoffmann (infancy onset) and Kugelberg-Welander (ages 1½–17). The gene for this single disease has been characterized and shoud lead to better understanding and treatment. This syndrome is primarily the province of pediatricians and family practitioners, with the adult PCP seeing adults who were diagnosed in childhood.

The final form of ALS, primarily lateral sclerosis, is the purely upper neuron form of the disease and is very rare.

Improved life expectancy of MND patients has been due entirely to better supportive care. Caring for these patients requires the same sensitivity as caring for terminally ill cancer patients. Depression is the rule, and caregiver and family stress is enormous. Hospice care is available to patients with an estimated life expectancy of 6 months. There are no medical management problems, aside from pneumonia, in these patients. They do not develop renal or liver failure, focal pain, confusional states, or the rest of the panoply of complications that lead to death in the usual medically ill patient. There are few medical encounters, therefore. As a result, the patient-family constellation may get lost in the medical system, with neither the neurologist nor the PCP having anything to offer. Support groups, medical access, and attention to emotional needs obviously are the highest priority.

MULTIPLE SCLEROSIS

Although uncommon, multiple sclerosis (MS) is nevertheless the most disabling neurologic disorder of young adults in the Western world. The name of the disease derives from the pathologic appearance of the cut brain, which reveals multiple sclerotic or scarred patches in the white matter. The disease is clearly autoimmune in nature, although not increased in frequency among patients with systemic autoimmune disorders such as rheumatoid arthritis, lupus erythematosus, or immune deficiency states. It affects women over men at a rate of 2 to 1 and initially develops between the third and fifth decades, peaking in onset at about age 30 (Table 11.4).

Table 11.4.   Multiple sclerosis

Uncommon; affects men and women
Episodic attacks or slow, chronic progression
Usually affects vision, gait, and bladder
Diagnosed with magnetic resonance imaging
Treatment should be via a neurologist

The epidemiology of MS holds the key to understanding its etiology, but it still has not yielded its secret despite decades of hypothesis testing. MS incidence increases with distance from the equator, in either direction, mostly as an association with climate. The incidence is determined by where the first 10–15 years were lived, so that children raised in the tropics who move to less temperate climates have a lower risk and vice versa. If a first-degree family member has MS, the risk is about 1–3%—small, but more than 15-fold greater than in the general population. Monozygotic twins have a 25% concordance rate, implying a strong genetic component.

MS produces a huge number of symptoms that are frequently dismissed early on by the patient's physicians. Fatigue and peculiar sensory symptoms such as tingling, aching, and numbness in distributions that are frequently nonphysiologic (meaning that they do not fit patterns of nerve or central nervous system disease) are common. Many patients with these symptoms, however, do not seek medical attention. The core symptoms that bring the patient to the doctor are problems with vision, coordination, balance, or bladder control. MS has a predilection for the spinal cord and optic nerves. When the disease affects the optic nerve, the condition is called optic neuritis (see Chapter 7) due to the inflammatory nature of the lesion. When the spinal cord is attacked in one place and affects most functions at one level, it is called a *transverse myelitis* (inflammation across the whole cord). The optic nerve lesion causes diminished color sensation and blurred vision out of one eye that cannot be corrected with lenses. With a severe attack or repeated attacks, vision may be lost, although this is uncommon. When the nerve is attacked near the termination in the retina (the optic disk), one sees the inflammation, which looks like papilledema, with the ophthalmoscope. More proximal lesions initially produce no fundus changes, but over time the disk becomes pale. Double vision occurs when upper brain stem disease causes weakness of extraocular muscles. Spinal cord involvement frequently affects bladder control and gait. The hallmark of the upper motor neuron or spastic bladder is the uninhibited contraction. The bladder, which is actually a smooth muscle under spinal cord and brain control, normally develops mild spasms when full, producing the urge to empty. When a patient has a spastic bladder, the contractions are excessively strong, producing the sense of urgency, and they develop at a very low capacity, producing a more frequent need to urinate than normal. Hence, patients develop frequency and urgency and note that they often have nocturia despite fluid restriction. The incontinence that occurs is generally large scale and is not to be confused with stress incontinence that is frequent after childbirth, in which women lose a few drops of urine with a cough or a sneeze. Patients with MS wet the floor and cannot compensate with a menstrual pad.

Gait dysfunction occurs from cerebellar involvement causing imbalance, corticospinal tract lesions causing spasticity, weakness, or all three. There may be problems almost anywhere in the central nervous system, so that one may encounter arm or leg weakness, clumsiness, speech alterations, and sensory changes. For unknown reasons, MS tends not to cause strokelike syndromes, so that hemiparesis, aphasia, apraxia, and homonymous field cuts are distinctly rare.

MS symptoms tend to develop over minutes to hours and, with the exception of optic neuritis, tend not to be painful at the lesion site, although the lesions may cause pain syndromes such as tic douloureux.

The clinical course of MS is categorized in two groups: the relapsing remitting variant and the chronic progressive form. In the former, patients develop symptoms that resolve. The chronic progressive form produces a progressive illness without remissions. Both forms are highly unpredictable in terms of prognostication in any particular case. Usually the relapsing remitting form transforms after several attacks to the progressive form.

Diagnosis of MS is usually straightforward with magnetic resonance imaging (MRI). The clinical diagnosis of MS rests on the old criteria that require two or more lesions separated in time and space, not explainable by the presence of any other condition, with a clear abnormality found on neurologic examination. The MRI has been a great help in diagnosing MS but is not without pitfalls. The brain MRI is positive in about 90% of cases and the MRI of the cervical cord enhances the yield still further, but about 5% of people believed to have MS have negative MRIs for reasons not yet explained. More problematic is the extreme sensitivity of the MRI, which can find T_2-enhancing patches in a very large percentage of people who do not have MS. These are usually read as ischemic vascular disease (but not stroke) or areas of demyelination and are found in diabetics, hypertensives, the elderly, migraineurs, and normals. Brain CT is not useful. Cerebrospinal fluid analysis is helpful in about 85% of cases, showing the presence of oligoclonal bands, which are antibodies directed at myelin, that are identifiable for many years after the last attack even as the illness appears to be quiescent. Immunoglobulin levels may be elevated as well. Glucose is normal. Protein is normal or mildly elevated. The cell count is normal in remission and shows a lymphocytosis, almost always under 100 cells per mm^3 in active disease. Myelin basic protein is elevated in active disease. Evoked responses (visual, auditory, and somatosensory) are used to demonstrate the presence of additional central nervous system lesions.

The diagnosis of MS should be made by a neurologist, as there are many considerations for the PCP that affect diagnostic possibilities: the psychosocial ramifications of living with an unpredictable illness, the concurrence of other neurologic disorders, the patient's tendency to embellish, distinguishing the emotional changes that may be reactive to the diagnosis or part of the illness, and management.

The most important factor to keep in mind in long-term management is kidney function. A small percentage of patients develop bladder-sphincter dyssynergia, which means that the normal yoking of bladder contraction and urethral sphincter relaxation is lost so that both may contract simultaneously, leading to urine reflux, hydronephrosis, and renal failure. For this reason, I strongly recommend that any MS patient with bladder involvement have regular consultations with a urologist.

Treatment of MS remains controversial. The U.S. Food and Drug Administration has approved three immune-directed therapies for relapsing remitting MS only. These are expensive and have a high incidence of intolerable side effects but do result in a mild reduction in disease progression. No treatment restores function. Many physicians use steroids to treat acute attacks. Some MS specialists use cyclophosphamide or azathioprine on a chronic basis. These interventions should be reserved for MS specialists. The important point about steroids is that they should never be used on a chronic basis, probably for less than a week after an acute attack, and only once a month for "maintenance." In the past, many MS patients were taking daily prednisone and years later paying the heavy price that comes with the drug, while their disease progressed anyway. The optic neuritis study group published the surprising results that prednisone given for a first attack of optic neuritis actually increased the chance of developing MS while intravenous methylprednisolone mildly decreased it.

Prognosis in MS is highly variable. Life expectancy is usually not shortened. About 60% of patients are independently ambulatory 15 years after a first attack. Younger-onset patients whose first attack resolves rapidly do quite well, as do patients who have little disability 5 years into the illness.

The common issue of pregnancy with MS should be discussed with a neurologist.

NORMAL PRESSURE HYDROCEPHALUS

Normal pressure hydrocephalus (NPH) is a much-discussed, presumably reversible dementing syndrome that is as rare as Jacob-Creutzfeldt disease, occurring in about 1 person per million per year. Although

NPH is billed as a dementing illness, few demented patients with hydrocephalus and a gait disorder reverse with shunting. The diagnosis of this disorder rests on clinical acumen acquired with experience that few neurologists or neurosurgeons have. There is no reliable diagnostic study. A good response to a lumbar puncture predicts a good response to shunting, but a poor response to a lumbar puncture does not predict a poor response to shunting.

NPH should be considered a gait disorder that may be associated with mild dementia and urinary urgency or incontinence.

SHY-DRAGER SYNDROME

Shy-Drager syndrome is another rare syndrome frequently discussed when parkinsonian patients faint. This eponym should be reserved for the parkinsonian patient who has no tremor and, without pressors, is unable to stand without fainting. Impaired bladder control is generally present as well.

CLINICAL PEARLS

- PD usually begins on one side and afflicts one side more than the other.
- NPH is extremely rare, probably about as common as Jacob-Creutzfeldt disease.
- Shy-Drager syndrome is also very rare.
- Head tremors are rarely due to PD.
- MRI is the best diagnostic test for MS.
- MS may develop in patients in late middle age.
- Optic neuritis is often part of MS but not always.

12

Neurologic Emergencies

There are few neurologic emergencies and all are uncommon. Historically, there have been only five: status epilepticus, epidural spinal cord compression, cerebral herniation, cerebellar hematoma, and monocular blindness (transient or persistent). The development of thrombolytic therapy for stroke in the first 3 hours, however, has made a "brain attack" a sixth emergency.

Status epilepticus is treated either in the emergency room or the intensive care unit of a hospital. The average primary care physician (PCP) should not have to deal with this problem without the assistance of skilled and knowledgeable personnel. Cerebral herniation occurs from expanding mass lesions in a patient who is comatose. This, too, is a hospital-based problem requiring the intervention of a neurosurgeon or a neurologist for management. Unlike the other emergencies, cerebral herniation, unless from a subdural or epidural hematoma, usually carries a bad prognosis from the underlying lesion even if the herniation itself is successfully treated. Cerebellar hematoma requires an emergency neurosurgical evaluation because edema may lead to brain stem compression with cranial neuropathies and coma that may reverse with early surgery. Loss of vision in one eye requires an evaluation for temporal arteritis.

STROKE

Ischemic (nonhemorrhagic) strokes can be treated with a thrombolytic drug within 3 hours of onset. If a patient awakens with a stroke, the stroke is assumed to be more than 3 hours old and therefore is untreatable. To be treated, however, the patient must go to a hospital that is prepared to administer tissue plasminogen activator (t-PA). The PCP should be aware of which hospitals in his or her area have a stroke team that provides this service and should have patients who might qualify go there directly without assessment in the PCP's office or in his or her own hospital. Time is of the essence and the 3-hour window of opportunity is not flexible. We know that at 3 hours there is more benefit than risk, and at 6 hours there is more risk than benefit, so every minute counts.

EPIDURAL SPINAL CORD COMPRESSION

Epidural spinal cord compression is the only neurologic emergency that often goes unrecognized until too late, leading to a disastrous outcome. It is also the main ambulatory neurologic emergency. About 5–10% of patients with cancer develop epidural metastases, which are tumors based in the vertebral body that grow posteriorly, emerging from the bone, and, no longer encased by a firm structure, simply expand up, down, and outward within the epidural space. Occasionally, an epidural metastasis is the presenting feature of the disease, and the patient is not known to harbor a malignancy until this point.

In most cases, the patient first develops a nagging, persistent pain in the back, localized to the involved thoracic vertebral bodies. Unlike most back pain, which is lumbosacral in origin, metastases tend to lodge in the thoracic vertebral bodies, although other regions may also be affected. The pain is initially of bone origin and does not radiate or cause neurologic symptoms. It may or may not be relieved or exacerbated by altered postures. Over a period of days or weeks, and occasionally over a period of only hours, the patient develops radicular pain and a sensation of tightness that feels like a belt or a girdle around the involved level. Examination at this point may reveal a mild sensory level, with pin and temperature sensations slightly reduced below the lesion. There might be mild spasticity, brisk or pathologic reflexes in the legs (positive Babinski reflexes, sustained clonus of the ankles, etc.), or diminished rectal tone. As the tumor further compromises the cord, weakness of both legs, possibly symmetric but not necessarily, develops along with numbness and urinary retention. Overflow incontinence frequently masks the bladder problem, and the diminished sensation keeps the patient from recognizing urinary dysfunction so that checking for postvoided bladder residua is very important.

The emergency nature of the situation derives from two observations. The first is that some patients dramatically worsen over hours, perhaps going to bed ambulatory and awakening paraplegic. The second is that recovery is inversely proportional to the severity of the deficit. A wheelchair-bound patient will likely remain wheelchair bound until death, which might be several months away. Ambulatory patients are likely to remain ambulatory. The quality of life issue for a terminally ill cancer patient is obvious: ambulatory and continent versus paraplegic and incontinent. Urgent or emergency magnetic resonance imaging (MRI) is the diagnostic test of choice when the index of suspicion is high.

STATUS EPILEPTICUS

Status epilepticus (SE) is an emergency because it can cause brain damage. It does so through two mechanisms. First, the repeated seizures may cause neuronal damage from the uncontrolled synchronous electrical discharges. Second, the repeated muscle contractions and diminished respiration during the seizures put a tremendous demand on the heart and also cause persistent acidosis and hypoxia. These factors may lead to a metabolic condition that is also toxic to the brain. Animal experiments with paralyzed animals whose electrolyte state, oxygen, and pH status were maintained revealed that persistent brain seizures still cause neuronal damage. Thus, paralyzing a seizing patient merely masks the problem and may lead to greater brain damage as the seizure continues unabated.

SE can be grouped into two broad categories of etiology: those with new structural or metabolic problems and those with a known seizure disorder and no new lesions. The latter almost invariably is due to acute discontinuation of anticonvulsant drugs but may also be due to drug abuse with cocaine, phencyclidine ("angel dust"), or amphetamines or to abrupt alcohol cessation. These patients are generally responsive to therapy instituted early.

New structural lesions such as strokes (ischemic or hemorrhagic), tumors, trauma, and infection (encephalitis or meningoencephalitis) carry a worse prognosis because there may be brain damage from the lesion as well as the seizures. The presence of SE does not by itself confer greater morbidity from the lesion. That is, one cannot assume that a stroke that induced SE causes a greater deficit than a stroke that did not.

The differential diagnosis for SE includes pseudoseizures, rigors with high fever, neuroleptic malignant syndrome, acute infection in an elderly patient with Parkinson's disease (PD), post–anoxic myoclonus, and decorticate or decerebrate posturing. As noted in Chapter 4 on epilepsy, pseudoseizures may be difficult to distinguish from organic seizures. They often last longer (organic seizures usually last under 2 minutes and almost never exceed 4) and are less vigorous, with more writhing and less tonic and clonic activity, less obtundation during the postictal state (more likely to show a response to painful stimuli), rare cyanosis or acidosis, and less likely presence of incontinence. Rigors, neuroleptic malignant syndrome, and fever in the elderly PD patient all look alike. The patient is usually obtunded with a varying level of responsiveness and stiffness and a variable degree of tremors, often occurring episodically. Usually the patient is not unconscious, as in SE, and the duration of the shaking and stiffening is very variable, often lasting several minutes at a time. Immediately after the attack, the patient is awake to some degree and capable of some voluntary movement. An electroencephalogram (EEG), if available, would show artifact and slowing but not epileptiform activity.

Posturing, either decorticate (legs extended and arms flexed with the fists near the chest) or decerebrate (legs extended and arms extended down to the hips), is caused by upper brain stem dysfunction and may also come in waves. These postures are tonic in nature and look like tonic seizures. The patient is comatose. They can be distinguished from seizures by their highly variable duration, their occurrence as a response to a noxious stimulation (e.g., suctioning or squeezing a nail bed), and their occurrence in someone comatose. The face and eyes are not involved, although gaze deviation may be present from the brain lesion that is causing the posturing. After resuscitation from a cardiopulmonary arrest, some patients have rapid, simple or repetitive sudden muscle jerks that are myoclonic. These can look like brief seizures.

MONOCULAR BLINDNESS

The most common cause of acute visual loss in one eye is atherosclerotic disease in the form of anterior ischemic optic neuropathy. Patients develop sudden painless loss of vision in one eye due to infarction. A second cause of visual loss is retinal artery infarction, generally from emboli, and a third is retinal venous infarction. Monocular blindness from temporal arteritis (TA) occurs on a vasculitic basis and is an emergency because the second eye is at high risk. Recovery from TA-induced blindness does not occur. No matter how high a steroid dose is used and no matter how soon it is instituted, blindness is permanent. Steroids, however, can save the good eye if instituted quickly. When TA is a consideration, prednisone, 100 mg, should be given, the erythrocyte sedimentation rate measured, and an ophthalmology consult or temporal artery biopsy obtained. History suggestive of TA includes headache and scalp tenderness, jaw claudication, chronic malaise, weakness, weight loss, or a history of polymyalgia rheumatica (persistent proximal muscle pain and tenderness) in a patient older than 60, and generally older than 70.

CEREBRAL HERNIATION

Cerebral herniation refers to the anatomic description of a brain displaced downward through the tentorium cerebri by a mass lesion in the hemispheres. As a result of downward herniation, pressure on the reticular activation system in the upper brain stem produces first stupor and then coma. When the herniation is lateralized, the onset of coma occurs in parallel with a third nerve palsy (dilated, fixed pupil, eye deviated outwards) as the brain squeezes the third nerve. This is accompanied by rapid breathing. With further unimpeded herniation, both pupils become dilated and fixed, coma deepens, more upper brain stem abnormalities occur, and the respiratory pattern slows and becomes irregular. Treatment is surgical, if possible. Dexamethasone is given if there is cerebral edema surrounding a tumor or an abscess. Steroids have been shown to have no benefit in reducing edema after a stroke or brain trauma. Hyperventilation causes a decline in blood carbon dioxide, leading to an immediate shrinkage of the normal brain and a reduction of intracranial pressure. Mannitol given at 1 g/kg similarly reduces the size of the normal brain, allowing more intracranial space for the mass. These are obviously only temporizing measures until a definite treatment—namely, evacuation of the mass and radiation therapy—is provided.

CEREBELLAR HEMORRHAGE

Hemorrhages in the cerebellum cause the sudden onset of limb or gait ataxia. There may be headache, but not always. Although the patient may appear perfectly alert and attentive, edema may develop, causing pressure on the brain stem. This induces cranial neuropathies or other brain stem deficits and an impaired level of consciousness. If these deficits persist for a few hours, they become permanent. There-fore, one has to prevent the problem or at least have the patient (and neurosurgeon) ready for emergency surgery as soon as lethargy sets in. When a patient is found to have an acute cerebellar stroke syn-drome, emergency computed tomography (CT) scan is required to evaluate for a possible hemorrhage. If a hemorrhage is found, a neu-rosurgeon needs to be apprised of the case.

Cerebellar infarcts are far less likely to cause similar problems and are more indolent in their expansion. On rare occasion the infarcted tissue may need to be removed. Steroids are frequently given in these situations but are of no benefit and are not recommended.

CLINICAL PEARLS

- Always check the bladder for postvoid residual in any patient suspected of spinal cord compression.
- Always consider spinal cord compression in any cancer patient with back pain and leg weakness, bladder problems, or walking problems.
- Spinal cord compression from metastatic cancer can progress over minutes.
- SE may cause brain damage even if the patient has completely normal metabolic parameters. Therefore, patients should be aggressively treated but not paralyzed unless an EEG is monitoring the seizure.
- The finding of cerebellar hemorrhage on a CT scan should trigger a neurosurgical consultation for possible hematoma evacuation.
- Early signs of cerebral herniation are declining level of consciousness and increasing respiratory rate.
- Myoclonus after an ischemic-hypoxic insult is a poor prognostic sign for recovery but does not require treatment unless it interferes with ventilation.

Appendixes

Appendix 1

The Neurologic Examination

The neurologic examination is of variable form and expands or contracts with the nature of the patient (and the expertise and interest of the examiner). There are several books devoted to examinations. There are books devoted even to parts of the examination, such as the mental status or the cranial nerve examination. There is even one book devoted entirely to interpreting the drawing of a clock! The minimum examination evaluates five modalities: mental state, cranial nerves, motor examination, sensory examination, and gait and station (posture and balance). An evaluation by a neurologist should include all these items for every patient, regardless of the symptoms.

THE BRIEFEST EXAMINATION

Independently, a colleague and I came up with the briefest examination we each could think of for the "neurologically challenged" physician. If a patient can hop on one foot with eyes closed, the chances are probably better than 90% that a neurologist would find no significant abnormalities on a formal examination.

MENTAL STATUS EXAMINATION

The mental status examination is often accomplished informally during the history taking. During this time one makes assessments of the patient's level of alertness, attention, intelligence, affect, memory, and other various functions. It is surprising, however, how often one can miss gross abnormalities of mental function by not testing certain functions in a formal routine fashion. For most patients this is probably not relevant and need not be done. Whenever a patient is admitted to the hospital, however, especially if it is because of a change in mental function, it is important that all significant aspects of mental functioning be tested, in part to point to a diagnosis and in part to provide a baseline from which to follow the patient's progress. There are obvious differences in certain aspects of the mental status examination between the assessments of the inpatient and the outpatient. Clearly, coma is not something one comes across in an outpatient setting, although on occasion a patient comes in stuporous. Level of alertness is probably the first thing that one can assess on observing a patient. In the hospital the patient might be asleep, so the amount of difficulty required to arouse the patient, how long it takes the patient to come to his or her senses, and whether the patient simply falls back to sleep while being assessed are all important factors that should be documented in the chart.

The patient in the office is usually quite alert. The attention that the patient is able to provide, however, is a very important characteristic that goes awry in demented and emotionally disturbed patients. The patient's affect, which is the mood the patient conveys, can be assessed. Frequently, one cannot interpret the patient's affect as "company manners" are on display, masking depression and anxiety because of the social stigma attached to letting down one's guard. In these cases, of course, the patient may need to be quizzed directly: "Are you feeling depressed, sad, blue?" "Are you more irritable than usual?" "Are people complaining that you are irritable and difficult to be around recently?" These may be markers for depression. Family members may need to be interviewed.

Orientation is a very crude mental anchor that should be accurate in all subjects, although normality depends on context. For example, a long-term nursing home patient may know neither the day of the week nor the date within the month, but should be aware of the month, year, and season. Most patients know where their doctor's office is located or the name of the doctor they are seeing, but occasionally, especially in the case of a nursing home resident who may be seeing a new doctor or several doctors, the exact name or the location of the doctor may not be known. The patient, however, should know that he or she is seeing the doctor and is not in a post office, a train station, or a church. It is surprising how often a patient who retains normal social graces can hide a significant level of dementia simply by being affable. Normal social intercourse requires very little in the way of knowledge and frequently relies on generalizations. For example, one can make comments about politicians or local sports teams without knowing a thing about what actually is happening.

Language function is very important in assessing dementia and confusional states. Aphasia is frequently an early sign of cortical dementias, particularly Alzheimer's disease (AD). Wernicke's aphasia, which is a fluent aphasia, is often mistaken for confusion. In this condition the patient shows few or no focal signs and babbles in a manner that seems superficially to make sense in that grammar appears to be normal, but no meaning is conveyed.

The patient's appearance and style of interaction should be noted. The patient who looks to a spouse for answers or who says "Huh?" after each question may be demented.

Language may be tested in five areas. One of these areas is naming, in which the patient is asked to give the name of fairly common body parts or objects around the room. All answers should be completely correct. When pointing to an eyebrow it is not correct for the patient to say "eyelid" or "eyelash"; it must be "eyebrow." If the patient's primary language is not English, then these answers should be given in the patient's native language, and the translator should be asked to state whether the answers were exactly correct. Several objects should be pointed to, not just two or three. All answers must be correct.

Reading, writing, repetition, and comprehension are the other four language functions tested. A patient should be asked to read something that requires a reasonable level of comprehension, such as newspaper headlines or introductory paragraphs from a magazine, and then be asked for content. Comprehension can be graded on a variety of levels. The normal individual can easily follow a three-step command. If the patient is incapable of doing this, then one can check for two-step or one-step commands. Repetition involves the patient repeating a phrase back exactly as stated. These can progress from simple statements such as "look at the cat" to more complex statements that are particularly difficult for aphasics such as, "The train came into the station over an hour late." (Aphasics have problems with short connecting words like *on*, *in*, *under*, and *over*, and tend to confuse them.) Writing, however, is probably the single most sensitive indicator of aphasia. When the patient does not have right arm weakness, he or she should be asked to write some sentences. The patient should be observed for grammatical and gross spelling errors. Language-disturbed patients leave out words, add extra curls onto letters, and make mistakes that are atypical of simple spelling errors.

Language fluency refers to the ease with which the patient speaks—specifically, how long the phrases are. Normal speech proceeds in the usual manner. Nonfluent speech consists of brief monosyllabic utterances produced with obvious effort.

Dysarthria is not to be confused with aphasia. Dysarthria is abnormally produced speech, the vocalized output of language. A sore tongue produces abnormal speech—hence dysarthria, not aphasia.

Constructional ability can be tested using the clock drawing and the intersecting pentagons. Sometimes these are abnormal in a way that points to a focal deficit, such as the clock that shows numbers only on the right-hand side, but more often the abnormalities are more consistent with a global derangement of thinking functions. In Parkinson's disease (PD) the numbers are frequently clustered near the middle, leaving a halo of unused space within the clock. Intersecting pentagons may show clumsy drawings but should show two five-sided figures that intersect appropriately. Other drawings, of course, also can be used to test the patient's function. Results must be interpreted in light of the patient's premorbid background. A professional artist is held to a higher standard than an eighth grade dropout who was never artistic.

Memory is tested for immediate, delayed, and remote stores. Remote functions involve questions such as "Who participated in World War II?" "Who was General Eisenhower?" or "How did John Kennedy die?" Immediate memory tests the patient's ability to register objects and recall them a few minutes later. One can further test an incorrect response by giving cues. If this is not sufficient, a "multiple choice" list should be provided in which one answer out of three or four is correct. Different dementing illnesses cause different memory problems. For example, in PD the patient may have difficulty with recall but actually has a memory trace imprinted in the brain so that a list jogs a correct answer. In AD or Wernicke-Korsakoff psychosis, however, no memory trace was made so that no correct answer can be gotten by providing appropriate hints.

The Mini-Mental State Examination is widely used and quite generally accepted. It provides a baseline for testing patients, although not as detailed as what is discussed above.

CRANIAL NERVE EXAMINATION

There are 12 cranial nerves, not all of which are clinically important. Testing the nerves is actually quite simple and fast. The first cranial nerve evaluates smell. This is rarely of importance in neurologic problems other than when the patient complains of abnormal smell or taste. Smell is frequently disrupted by significant head trauma. It can also be affected, of course, by upper respiratory infection, cigarette smoking, and a variety of other things that affect the nasal passages. In actual clinical practice, this is rarely useful to test.

The eyes are innervated by cranial nerves 2, 3, 4, and 6. One tests visual fields via confrontation. That is, one can simply put one's arms roughly halfway between the patient and oneself and, using one's own peripheral vision as the presumptive norm, test the patient by raising one or two fingers. When the visual fields are not important, it can be done by testing only the upper and lower outer quadrants with both eyes open. In cases in which each eye needs to be tested, then one eye is covered. The doctor should close the opposite eye and have the patient stare eye-to-eye and test as above, again using one's own visual field as the norm. Funduscopic and pupillary examinations are straightforward. It is always important to keep in mind that cataract surgery or other trauma to the eye may alter the pupils or lids, making their response, or

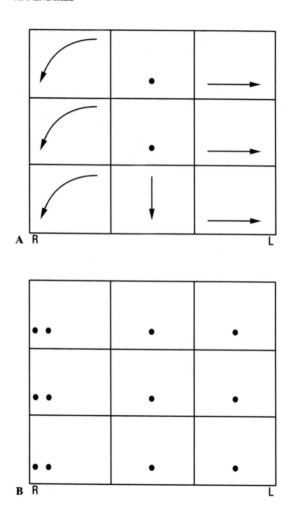

A R   L

B R   L

lack thereof, of no clinical use. Eye movements are often complex when disordered. Eye movements are checked by having the patient follow a moving object. Looking up is important but commonly decreases with normal aging. The best way to keep track of abnormal eye movements is to attempt to write them down. Figure A1.1 is a tic-tac-toe drawing that illustrates how one keeps track of eye movements. The middle box shows the eyes in primary position; to the left and to the right would be the eye movements when looking right or left; the upper row would be looking up in the middle, to the right or left; and the lower row shows down-gaze to the right, left, and middle. One can then graph how the eyes move if they are in any way abnormal. For example, with right-beating nystagmus, on looking to the right, one would put an arrow pointing to the right in the right box. If the eyes were normal in primary position—that is, with the eyes straight ahead—one would just put in zero or nothing at all. If there were down-beating nystagmus in primary position, one would put a down arrow. The length of the arrow would be proportional to the severity of the nystagmus. When one encounters inner ear dysfunction, there is frequently rotary nystagmus. In this case the eye does not beat to the left or right but rotates in a clockwise or counterclockwise fashion. This is indicated on the grid with a curving arrow, again keeping size proportional to the severity or the amplitude of the movements. One can also use the grid for keeping track of diplopia if the patient complains of double vision. One should then ask whether the objects are side-by-side, on top of each other, or on a diagonal, and roughly how far apart they are. One then notes this in the appropriate tic-tac-toe box. If the abnormal eye movements can be more easily described in terms of which eye muscles are involved, then that should be recorded. Using this method of tracking the eye movements, however, one does not have to try to recall, perhaps inaccurately,

◄ **Figure A1.1.** A. This grid indicates counterclockwise nystagmus looking to the right, left beating nystagmus looking left, and down beating nystagmus looking down. B. This grid indicates horizontal diplopia looking to the right. Arrows indicate the direction and severity of nystagmus. Dots indicate the visual image perceived.

what was observed, and one does not have to try to interpret it on the spot. But with results in hand, one can call an appropriate authority and describe in detail what was seen, allowing the expert to interpret the findings and come to an accurate diagnosis.

The fifth cranial nerve is evaluated by testing sensation on the face and the muscles of mastication. Clinically, the fifth nerve is rarely affected. The seventh nerve is very often affected in neurologic problems and is thus probably the most important cranial nerve for most neurologic problems. One tests fifth nerve function by asking the patient to raise the eyebrows, to close the eyes tightly, to smile, and sometimes to contract the platysma muscle. Upper motor neuron lesions—that is, those in the hemisphere—cause weakness that is below the eyebrow, whereas lower motor neuron weakness, such as with a Bell's palsy, causes weakness of the whole face, including the frontalis muscle. With hemispheric seventh nerve palsies, patients frequently can contract their face if they laugh spontaneously, but this does not occur with a forced laugh. With a Bell's palsy, this dissociation does not occur. The eighth nerve tests hearing and vestibular function. One can test vestibular function in a number of ways, including caloric testing, which is often somewhat difficult in the office. The Barany mentioned in Chapter 2 on dizziness is another approach. The ninth and tenth nerves subserve sensation in the pharynx and the gag reflex. With the exception of brain stem lesions, such as a brain stem stroke or a brain stem tumor, this is less clinically useful than is often thought. It is common for doctors and nurses to "test" whether a patient can swallow by looking for a gag reflex. This actually has little relationship to the patient's ability to swallow. Many patients have a perfectly normal gag reflex yet aspirate, and many people who swallow normally have no gag reflex at all. The abnormality that is useful for assessment is an asymmetric gag, in which the uvula deviates to one side. It deviates to the working side as the weak side fails to contract as strongly.

The eleventh cranial nerve innervates the shoulder shrug and the sternomastoid muscles, which turn the head. It is frequently affected by strokes. The twelfth cranial nerve protrudes the tongue and is frequently abnormal after strokes. One can remember that the protruded tongue deviates to the weak side by recalling how the tongue is protruded. Muscles only contract. The tongue protrudes because the contracting tongue muscles are very posterior in the hypopharynx and basically "push" the tongue out. This is the exact same mechanism that protrudes the jaw. The pterygoid muscles contract, but in doing so the upper jaw remains stationary and the lower jaw is "pushed" out as the attachment between the two structures shortens with the muscle contraction. When one side is weak, it is not "pushed" out and the result is like paddling a canoe. The canoe turns toward the side not being paddled or, in this case, being pushed. This is the weak side.

In short, the main concern in evaluating cranial nerves is that two sides should be symmetric. Asymmetry suggests a cranial neuropathy.

MOTOR EXAMINATION

The motor examination begins with an observation of the patient's musculature, looking for wasting and fasciculations. This is not always relevant but must be performed when assessing for weakness or neuropathy. The examiner should pay attention to excessive or diminished spontaneous movements. Is the patient akinetic or trembling in the resting position? Akinesia, of course, is a hallmark of parkinsonism. In general this is not important, but in the elderly it can be very important. Is the patient moving excessively and fidgeting, or is he or she not moving enough? One should consider the patient's facial expression. Does it look mask-like? In parkinsonism the facial expression is usually depressed or mildly angry. Is the patient blinking at a normal rate? If there is a tremor at rest, one may see it in the jaw, head, fingers, hands, or feet. In most cases it is obvious and the patient draws attention to it. I then check for pronator drift. This is done by having the patient extend the arms parallel to the ground, palms up. Pronator drift is a cortical spinal tract sign in which the affected arm drifts slightly downward and pronates. That is, the radial aspect of the arm starts to tilt up and the ulnar down. With a parietal or sensory defect, the arm frequently goes up and out. The eyes are closed during this maneuver, which takes about 10 seconds. I then ask the patient to touch his or her nose with a finger. This provides evidence of ataxia. The examiner can have the patient touch his or her finger, looking for overshoot, in which the patient consistently tries to reach beyond the finger, or past pointing, in which the patient is consistently off to one side of the target. These are cerebellar abnormalities. One also looks for a breakdown in the smoothness of the arm movement. Rapid alternating movements or dysdiadochokinesia is a measure of dexterity and is most commonly seen with cortical spinal tract abnormalities, but also with parkinsonism and cerebellar disorders. The internist or generalist really needs simply to document that there is an abnormality. Later, one can go back and try to figure out where the abnormality is within the nervous system. Tone is checked by having the patient relax and then the arms, legs, and neck are passively moved. This is generally of importance in gait disorders or in syndromes of clumsiness in which one is looking for evidence of cortical spinal tract disease, such as cervical myelopathies, which occur in multiple sclerosis and cervical spondylosis. The best way to check for spasticity in the knees is to have the patient relax in a supine position and then quickly raise the upper leg, grabbing just above the knee. The normal response, if the patient is relaxed, is for the heel to drag across the examining table. A spastic response would be for the lower leg to come up with the upper leg, possibly even jerking a few times. Spasticity is a rate-dependent reflex. The faster one moves the joint, the greater the increase in tone so that in a spastic leg, one can usually move the knee joint slowly without encountering much resistance. But if one moves it quickly, it suddenly stops before giving way again ("clasp-knife" response).

Strength testing is probably the most important aspect of the motor examination. On routine testing, one does not need to know the names of all the muscles. One can simply say that the proximal arms, elbows, or wrist extensors are weak, if they are. In the normal grading system used among neurologists, 5 represents normal strength. A 4 is subnormal but not as weak as a 3. A 3 means that a patient can only overcome gravity but not minimal resistance. A 2 indicates strength that cannot overcome gravity so that one can move a limb laterally but not up and down. A 1 reflects only a flicker of movement, and a 0 is complete paralysis. Most patients with weakness have a 4. When using this system, one should keep in mind the norm for the patient under evaluation. An 85-year-old frail person obviously does not have the strength of a younger, robust patient, so that a 5 for an older person would be a 4 for a younger one. Four or less indicates pathology. It is common for patients to be unable to be tested because of pain or ankylosis of a joint. In these cases, one should record what the minimum strength was but that accurate testing was precluded by pain.

Reflexes are important primarily for symmetry. Reflexes are somewhat position dependent and also vary with the patient's level of anxiety, so that one may find different reflexes at different times in the same patient. It is common for some reflexes to be absent in normal people. This is frequently the case in the arms in young people. It is also common for young women in particular to have two or three beats of clonus at the ankle. This, too, is not pathologic, although it would be in an older man. In the standard reflex grading, 0 is an absent reflex, 1 is a minimal reflex obtained with or without reinforcement, 2 is normal, 3 is brisk but not pathologic, and 4 reflects unsustained clonus, which is less than five beats after the initial hammer tap. Five is sustained clonus, meaning five beats or more. One then records the response to the Babinski maneuver. A positive reflex is pathologic, except in early childhood. A classic positive response involves fanning of the toes in extension with the big toe going up. When one repeats the Babinski maneuver, one often finds that the reflex changes. Any up movement of the toe, however, with the initial movement being the one that is recorded, is abnormal. There are a variety of ways of eliciting pathologic reflexes of equal significance to the Babinski. One can stroke the lateral aspect of the foot, run one's knuckles down the tibia, or grasp the Achilles tendon firmly.

SENSORY EXAMINATION

The sensory examination is the least reliable part of the neurologic examination because it is based on the patient's response and not on the observations of the doctor. It is most important to confirm symmetry of light touch and pinprick and to check whether a peripheral neuropathy may be present. One, of course, has certain indications of the possibility of nerve disease from the deep tendon reflex responses. If they are absent, one should be suspicious for a peripheral neuropathy. If reflexes are asymmetric, one should look for a pinched nerve. In performing the sensory examination, I generally touch the feet, hands, and face with a light object (frequently just with my finger). One can also include the trunk. I then repeat this with a pin. Position sense may be crucial in assessing gait abnormalities, as position sense impairment has a major impact on how one walks. If gait abnormality is not being considered and the patient has no other symptoms or signs to suggest the peripheral neuropathy, it can be left out. Assessing for peripheral neuropathy can be done quite quickly by simply marching a disposable pin up the leg from the foot. If the patient reports that the pin gets sharper above a certain point, that would be strong evidence for a neuropathy and might be confirmed by similarly testing the other leg. Diffuse peripheral neuropathies always manifest in the feet before the hands so that the hands need not be tested if the feet are normal. Sensory abnormalities due to problems in the cortex of the brain involve "higher" perceptions involving integration of information. One can trace numbers in the palm (graphesthesia) or stimulate both sides of the body at the same time to see if sensation on one side is extinguished.

Further testing might include vibratory sensation (although this is frequently diminished in normal aging). Cold and hot sensation should provide the same distribution of abnormalities as pin, because pin and temperature are carried by the same pathways within the central nervous system. And, finally, if one suspects nerve root compression or a nerve abnormality, one should test the appropriate part of the body in a more detailed fashion, trying to map out the area of sensation that is affected.

It is often not understood that all of these abnormalities exist across a spectrum of severity. In most peripheral neuropathies the patient has not lost sensation completely but has suffered an impairment. A sensory abnormality can be described along the continuum starting with normal and can be compared to wearing very fine surgical gloves; wearing thicker, disposable, nonsterile, nonsurgical gloves; and then wearing rubber dishwashing gloves. Obviously, with surgical gloves sensation is not normal but not terribly impaired. As one progresses up to the thicker, coarser types of gloves, the sensation is successively diminished. Thus, patients often experience a pin as feeling somewhat sharp in the toes but sharper in a more proximal region. The pin feels relatively dull distally. This notion of a spectrum of deficit severity also holds for isolated nerve root impingements and even more so for abnormalities of the central nervous system.

Patients may experience abnormal sensations in affected areas. Even though they may have diminished sensation, a pinprick or light touch may be painful. Patients may describe a sunburn-like sensation with diabetic neuropathy, for example. Nevertheless, their discrimination ability is diminished as a result of their peripheral neuropathy. The areas that are affected either with dysesthesia, which are abnormal sensations such as pain with touch or numbness, should be mapped out in some crude model drawn on the chart so that it can be compared with a textbook for finding the distribution and localizing the abnormality.

GAIT AND STATION EXAMINATION

The final portion of the neurologic examination pertains to gait and station. This is discussed in detail in Chapter 5. Patients are observed for posture as they sit in a chair and as they sit on the examining table where there is no back support. There may be a tendency for the patient to start falling backward or off to one side. This is abnormal and should be noted. The patient should be observed walking, preferably without any assistive device. One can then just assess briefly whether the patient walks normally or not. Is there an asymmetry to the arm swing? Is the base normal? The feet should be at shoulder length or less apart. Sometimes the gait is overly narrow, as occurs in spasticity, or too far apart, as with midline cerebellar degeneration. Does the patient appear to be unsteady? This is usually most obvious on turning.

ABBREVIATED EXAMINATIONS

The above is a rather complete neurologic examination and is generally performed by a neurologist on every new patient. In the office of a generalist, the parts of the neurologic examination that should be performed at the first office visit really depend on the patient. In a young, healthy patient the examination can be minimal, but certain parts should be documented as a baseline. In the elderly, a Mini-Mental State Examination should be obtained because it provides insight into possible early dementia with all its ramifications. For a young person coming in without a neurologic complaint, there is probably no benefit to a mental status examination beyond what is observed in routine history taking. Cranial nerve testing can probably be limited to looking for facial asymmetry. If the patient has a problem with eye movements, the patient undoubtedly complains of double vision, blurred vision, or some other problem. It may be useful to look at pupillary size because Horner's syndromes are fairly common and should be documented at baseline before the patient develops any further complaint where the presence of a new Horner's syndrome might be a crucial finding. The motor examination can be limited to looking for clumsiness with rapid arm movements and deep tendon reflexes. A brief sensory examination should be documented and the patient should be observed walking. In the elderly, tone and gait assume more importance as parkinsonism becomes more common.

PRINCIPLES OF LOCALIZATION

The job of a neurologist is to answer two questions when there is a neurologic problem, usually in the following order: where is the problem and what is the problem? One hundred years of clinical observation has led to the current neurologic examination and its interpretation. The principles of localization are actually much simpler than most physicians believe. These are based, of course, on neuroanatomy, which is incredibly complicated. (To paraphrase Dr. Robert Joynt, every part of the nervous system is connected to every other part and unfortunately many of these places and connections have names.) Clinically relevant neuroanatomy for the primary care physician (and even for most neurologists) is actually surprisingly simple.

Anatomy

- The hemisphere of the brain (portions above the tentorium cerebelli) connects to the opposite side of the body.
- The brain stem (midbrain, pons, medulla) and cerebellum connect to the same side of the face and opposite side of the body (almost 100% true).
- The spinal cord has a diameter about the size of your pinkie, so that small lesions may produce large deficits.

Principles

The one umbrella principle in neurology, as in all medicine, is the law of parsimony: One explanation is better than two.

- Abnormalities of face, arm, and leg on one side must arise from a lesion above the brain stem.
- The principle of crossed findings: If an abnormality occurs on one side of the face and the other side of the body, the lesion must be in the brain stem. Because motor tracts cross in the lower medulla and sensory tracts cross in the spinal cord, all fiber tracts in the brain stem go to or from the opposite side of the body. The cranial nerve nuclei, however (except cranial nerve IV, which is clinically irrelevant), serve the same side of the head. So, for example, a lesion at the level of the facial nerve on the left affects the left face and fiber tracts that are crossed, serving the right side of the body. Thus, facial weakness on one side and body weakness on the other must be caused by a left–brain stem process.
- Whenever the pupils or eye movements are affected (except bilateral gaze deviation), the lesion is in the brain stem.
- Bilateral leg problems are due to myopathy, neuropathy, or a spinal cord process.

- Bilateral arm and leg problems are in the cervical cord, if not from a neuropathy or myopathy.
- Speech and vision problems must arise from abnormalities above the spinal cord.
- Changes in language, memory, thinking, mood, attention, or other higher mental functions are always due to a process above the brain stem, usually in the cortex.
- A writing sample is the most sensitive indicator of aphasia. A signature is not sufficient. One or more complete sentences should be requested.
- Tremors always worsen with anxiety, fatigue, and exercise.
- Any patient with new bilateral leg weakness or spasticity requires a bladder evaluation (usually a postvoid residual measurement is adequate).
- The best way to test for dysphagia is to have the patient swallow a small amount of water. Gag reflex testing is a poor predictor of swallowing.
- Deep tendon reflexes vary with anxiety, posture, and degree of relaxation.
- When testing position sense, make sure the patient's digit is relaxed. Hold the digit on the sides.

Neurologic Tests

The most commonly ordered types of neurologic tests are imaging studies (computed tomography [CT] and magnetic resonance imaging [MRI]) and tests of physiology (electroencephalogram [EEG] and electromyogram [EMG]). Other tests, such as single photon emission computed tomography (SPECT), nuclear brain scans, and positron emission tomography, combine imaging with physiology, pharmacology, and biochemistry. Tests of body fluids are also important.

Although it is obvious that one should have a reasonable differential diagnostic list in mind before ordering a test, or at least a localization for the neurologic dysfunction, too often virtually any neurologic complaint triggers a brain CT scan and, until recently, an EEG. In my own community, a neurologist often obtained brain CT scans in advance of seeing patients for the first time! Aside from the obvious waste in this process, a patient occasionally has an abnormality identified on a CT scan, but the abnormality has nothing to do with the symptoms or signs found on examination (e.g., the elderly patient with a coincidental meningioma or old, clinically silent stroke).

MAGNETIC RESONANCE IMAGING

Imaging studies are obtained to evaluate the possibility of a structural abnormality. For most disorders, MRI is more sensitive than CT scanning. MRI does not involve radiation and has no complications. Moreover, there are no allergic reactions to the dye used for contrast-enhanced MRI.

MRI provides amazingly detailed images of the nervous system with an accuracy undreamed of even in the late 1980s. It is based on perturbations in the electric field induced by electromagnetic waves produced by an extremely powerful magnet. The only technical contraindications to its use are the presence of magnetic material in the patient (generally caused by shrapnel or metal shards from metal shops) or a pacemaker. Dental fillings and artificial joints are not contraindications. Because of claustrophobia, a fair percentage of patients cannot tolerate the MRI apparatus unless medicated. Most patients can be sufficiently sedated with a benzodiazepine, as long as they have a ride home after the test. (Benzodiazepines are generally very safe when taken orally. I generally prescribe 5–10 mg of diazepam taken about 2 hours before testing, with further doses to be allowed as needed.)

Principles

MRI provides the best imaging available for the brain. Its resolution is determined by the strength of the magnetic field. Thus, with technologic advances, even finer resolution is possible in the future. Most MRI research, however, is centered on the development of faster and better analyses of data that are already being generated. Important developments have included magnetic resonance angiography (MRA), magnetic resonance venography (MRV), and functional MRI (fMRI). MRA and MRV permit visualization of blood flow without the use of an arterial or venous dye load, and fMRI permits imaging based on metabolism so that brain regions that are metabolically active are more intense than those that are not. This technique can be used for testing brain functions, such as memory and language, and is useful as a research device. Its main clinical indication is for localizing epileptic foci for surgery. It is not yet available at most centers.

The major problem with MRI is its extreme sensitivity. Routine MRIs frequently pick up spots that have no clear meaning. Many of these spots are called *unidentified bright objects* (UBOs). Much effort has gone into identification of UBOs because they can be strokes, areas of demyelination, cerebrospinal fluid accumulations

**Table A2.1.   Computed tomography (CT) vs.
magnetic resonance imaging (MRI)**

CT is cheaper and more easily available
MRI is more sensitive for most conditions
MRI is sometimes overly sensitive
Claustrophobic patients require sedation for MRI
MRI cannot be performed in patients with ferromagnetic metals or a
  pacemaker
CT shows bone and blood more clearly

due to arteriolar shrinkage, or transient images of unknown significance. For example, in a clinical pathologic correlation (CPC) I did for the *New England Journal of Medicine*, the MRI showed a patchy region in the occipital white matter that was not, I thought, relevant to the case. Fortunately, I got the CPC correct and added, for good measure, that there was an unrelated stroke in the occipital lobe. For whatever reason, the brain was normal where the MRI lesion was, and neither the neuropathologist nor the neuroradiologist at one of the world's premier hospitals had an explanation. We shrugged our shoulders and called it a UBO. Unfortunately, at other times, a collection of UBOs is ominously indicative of either cerebrovascular disease or demyelinating disease.

COMPUTED TOMOGRAPHY VS. MAGNETIC RESONANCE IMAGING

There are logistic and technical reasons for choosing one imaging technique over another. CT scanning is cheaper and much more readily available. Most American hospitals have CT machines and testing can usually be done emergently. CT scans can be performed on claustrophobic patients and those with pacemakers and magnetic objects in their body (all metals, magnetic or not, however, distort the image; this only occurs when the metal is in the plane of the picture). Patients on ventilators can have a CT scan but usually not an MRI (Table A2.1).

CT scans are better for imaging acute blood than MRI. Therefore, a CT scan may be a more useful test than MRI in the emergency evaluation of a stroke patient who might receive tissue plasmogen activator (t-PA) or anticoagulation. MRI is considerably more sensitive for picking up intraparenchymal abnormalities, but it is less specific in its findings.

SINGLE PHOTON EMISSION COMPUTED TOMOGRAPHY

SPECT uses a radioactive substance to produce images of the brain. Currently, the only labeling substance commercially available in the United States is ^{99m}Tc HMPAO (technetium hexamethyl propyl-emamine-oxime), which provides a CT-type image of cerebral blood flow. Because blood flow parallels metabolism, ^{99m}Tc HMPAO provides direct information about blood flow and indirect information on metabolism. Current resolution (6–9 mm, using the best 1998 equipment) is at about the level of the original brain CT scans of the 1970s. SPECT is thus relatively crude.

SPECT scans have limited indications, although they can be very helpful in diagnosing dementias. Alzheimer's disease (AD) shows a characteristic decreased activity in both temporal-parietal regions. Pick's disease shows bifrontal hypometabolism, whereas multi-infarct or vascular dementia shows multifocal regions of diminished activity. SPECT scans can also be used to demonstrate reduced blood flow that indicates ischemic brain disease. Thus, a SPECT scan may reveal a stroke before the CT scan is positive or may reveal an underperfused brain that has had a recent transient ischemic attack. SPECT scans may also show "cold" spots, which are seizure foci—hypometabolic most of the time and hypermetabolic during a seizure. SPECT also illustrates abnormal metabolic activity and blood flow in brain tumors and adjacent regions.

The problem with SPECT is that, with the possible exception of AD, abnormalities are seen better with other tests. Even in AD, the abnormalities do not generally appear early. SPECT helps answer the question of how to diagnose a clearly present dementia but not whether the patient is demented or not.

SPECT will become more useful as new ligands are released that permit imaging of different neurotransmitter systems in the brain. Currently in testing are ligands that label the dopamine transporter, a protein that provides information on the status of dopamine-containing cells. Ultimately, this ligand may permit diagnosis, in a subclinical stage, of Parkinson's disease and other related disorders. With other ligands, we may be able to diagnose and monitor progression of a variety of brain disorders, both neurologic and psychiatric. For now, SPECT has more promise than immediate applicability.

CAROTID ULTRASOUND

Duplex carotid ultrasonography provides an image of the carotid artery as well as data on peak flow velocity, thus producing two separate sets of data on carotid stenosis. These data are personnel-dependent, so different laboratories may produce different results.

Carotid ultrasound is an extremely useful screening test for carotid stenosis because it is risk-free and easily tolerated. An insonation device is placed on the neck and angled in various directions. When the device is used effectively, results are reproducible. However, few surgeons proceed with an operation on the basis of an ultrasound exam. The standard angiogram is still the gold standard, although some surgeons find combined results of MRA and carotid duplex sufficient to proceed with endarterectomy.

This test is useful in any patient with transient ischemic attack or minor stroke who is a candidate for surgery and had the event in the carotid vascular supply. This test should not be performed to evaluate vertebral-basilar disease and is not indicated in the evaluation of dizziness of any type or fainting.

PHYSIOLOGIC TESTS

Electromyography

The EMG examination is only mildly uncomfortable, except for patients who are needle-phobic. For patients who have a phobia for

Table A2.2.   Electromyogram

Useful in evaluating neuropathies and myopathies
Very useful for diagnosing nerve entrapments
Very useful for diagnosing myopathies
Useful for diagnosing neuropathies and evaluating severity
Quality dependent on tester
Expensive

needles, one should ascertain in advance whether nerve conduction studies alone would be helpful. If not, the whole test should be aborted. The electric stimulations, described below, are mildly unpleasant but last only one-twentieth to one-tenth of a second per shock. Few patients have difficulty handling this. The EMG hurts a bit because a fine needle is inserted into a muscle, not a nerve (Table A2.2).

The standard EMG consists of two parts: a nerve conduction study and the EMG itself. These are generally considered together under the single rubric *EMG*. The EMG is useful in cases of nerve and muscle disorders, including nerve entrapments.

The nerve conduction study also has individual components. Motor nerves are tested by stimulating over distal and proximal points in a motor nerve. The response is measured by electrodes placed over a muscle innervated by the nerve. The EMG machine records the time taken from application of the stimulus to contraction of the muscle. This is called the *latency*. The machine also records the amplitude of the motor response. The nerve is then stimulated again at a proximal point and the same parameters are recorded. By measuring the distance between the points of stimulation, one can calculate the velocity of the impulse between the points. In demyelinating neuropathies, such as diabetes, the conduction velocity is slow because the speed of conduction is maintained by the myelin sheath. In axonal neuropathies, where the myelin sheath is intact but the axon degenerates, velocity is maintained but the amplitude of the response is reduced because fewer nerve fibers trigger fewer muscle fibers to contract.

The sensory nerve study measures the sensory nerve's response by stimulating and recording over the nerve. The amplitude and latency are recorded. The problem with sensory nerve recording is that recordings are only possible on a routine basis from the foot and hand, and patients with clinically minor neuropathies often have no response to nerve stimulation. It is overly sensitive.

Other nerve studies include the H-reflex, which is an electric analog of the ankle reflex, and the F wave. The F wave records the time required for an electric stimulus to travel proximally to the spinal cord and then back down to a distal muscle, causing contraction. When electric shocks are applied to a motor nerve, the stimulus travels in both directions. The F wave only records the later response. This is very helpful for conditions such as Guillain-Barré syndrome, in which the disease is patchy and multifocal. The F wave test allows for evaluation of the whole nerve, not just a distal segment.

The EMG requires a needle to be inserted into a muscle. No electric stimulus is applied. The physician interprets the electric pattern on an oscilloscope screen with the muscle at rest and under voluntary contraction. The various abnormalities of these patterns provide information as to whether this process is acute (weeks old) or chronic (months to years old). Testing muscles with different innervations can help determine whether the process is in the distribution of a single nerve root, a group of roots, or a nerve, or is part of a diffuse pattern.

The quality of the EMG depends enormously on the ability of the physician doing the test. Although there is a society that regulates the quality of those who pass special competency exams in EMG, any neurologist or physiatrist can perform these tests, whether sanctioned by this group or not. Because EMG is an expensive test that is well reimbursed, it is one of the only ways for doctors in these two fields, which are not procedure oriented, to gain economic ground with their more procedurally oriented colleagues. In fact, it is hard to pursue a private neurology or physiatry practice and stay afloat economically without doing EMGs. Unfortunately, this means that a large number of EMGs are not competently performed. Thus, it is important to know the experience and skill with EMG of the physician doing the test. If the physician is certified by the American Board of Electrodiagnostic Medicine or has a certificate of Advanced Qualifications in Neurophysiology, the patient can feel comfortable. If the physician is not certified, he or she may still be very competent, but one must be skeptical. Keep track of the reports and see how well the results are borne out by the unfolding clinical events (e.g., EMG agrees with the MRI or surgical results, EMG at local office agrees with a repeat performed at a university laboratory). Nerve conduction studies are often performed by technologists and are much less subject to errors of interpretation. The needle EMG must be performed by a physician.

Electroencephalogram

Like the EMG, EEG can be a useful test if performed at a good lab for the correct reasons. Also like EMG, many EEGs are not useful. The EEG is mainly useful in the evaluation of epilepsy. It can also be extremely helpful for early diagnosis of herpes simplex encephalitis, for diagnosing Jacob-Creutzfeldt disease late in the course, and in discriminating organic mental states from primary psychiatric conditions. The American Academy of Neurology has opined that EEG is not a useful test for evaluating headaches (Table A2.3).

Aside from diagnosing epilepsy, EEG is rarely used to diagnose other conditions. The EEG is usually normal in early to moderate AD and therefore is not helpful for diagnosing this disorder or distinguishing it from other dementing disorders. The EEG may be helpful in categorizing epilepsy into generalized or focal and in determining how active a seizure focus is. The EEG can be helpful in investigating the common problem of unwitnessed loss of consciousness, after which the patient recalls nothing from immediately before the attack. Statistically these spells are likely to be due to cardiac arrhythmias or other hypotensive disorders but are occasionally seizure-induced. In the past EEGs were obtained on a regular basis to monitor seizure control, but there is little need for this. Once seizures have been diagnosed, the only further roles for the EEG are for (1) diagnosing "spells" that are different from the known seizure and may represent

Table A2.3.   Electroencephalogram

Useful for diagnosing seizures
Useful in evaluating unwitnessed loss of consciousness
Not for headache evaluation
Used to evaluate risk of stopping anticonvulsants
Not required on a routine basis
Quality dependent on tester

a new seizure type or something nonepileptic, (2) assessing the likelihood of a recurrent seizure once anticonvulsant drugs are stopped, (3) looking for subclinical seizures to explain behavioral alterations, and (4) to look for new seizure foci. Most of these reasons should involve a neurologist. Once a patient is stable, there is probably no reason for repeating the EEG except out of habit.

One very real question is whether an EEG is necessary at all for a patient who had a witnessed seizure. The decision to start an anticonvulsant is, after all, a clinical decision. Most neurologists recommend that an EEG be obtained after a first seizure. The rationale is that the EEG may diagnose the seizure type and thus provide information on prognosis and the choice of medication. It may also reveal subclinical epileptiform activity. In fact, results that alter therapy or provide prognostic information are uncommon. Missing this information by not ordering a noninvasive, inexpensive test, however, would be considered negligent. The standard procedure is to obtain an EEG. A brain-imaging study is always the most important diagnostic test for evaluating an adult who has had a first seizure.

In children with petit mal seizures (not to be confused with complex partial or temporal lobe seizures), frequent EEGs may be necessary to monitor drug response because the typical seizure may not be appreciated by the child or the physician and an EEG may reveal huge numbers of clinically undetectable seizures (see Chapter 4 on epilepsy).

One problem with the EEG is that, like the electrocardiogram (ECG), it provides only a brief record (30–45 minutes) of brain activity. Seizures are very infrequent events. Interictal spike and sharp waves are more frequent but still not common. True seizure foci are frequently missed due to sampling problems, and an epileptic may have a normal EEG. For some patients, especially those with spells of an unclear nature, a closed-circuit television (TV) EEG is very useful. Patients are monitored for 8 hours a day for up to 3 days, with a continuous EEG running on one half of a split screen TV and the patient on video camera on the other half. The patient, if capable, presses an "event" button when sensing a "spell." A correlation between the video of the patient and the EEG can then be made using the TV EEG and the actual paper tracing. These tests are very likely to confirm or exclude a diagnosis of epilepsy.

EEGs are too often over-read, with normal records read as abnormal, and often end with one of the following disconcerting pronouncements: "Clinical correlation required," "Cannot exclude convulsive tendency," or "Repeat EEG suggested." Some readers of EEGs have a huge, murky, gray zone of interpretations that leaves the primary care physician further out on a limb even after the test. The trick is to order an EEG only when necessary and then have it interpreted by a competent, conservative electroencephalographer. As with EMG interpretation, most neurologists reading this test have not passed examinations to demonstrate competence. Most, if not all, epilepsy experts request previous EEG records on their new patients and not the EEG reports because of discrepant interpretations.

Cerebrospinal Fluid

Cerebrospinal fluid (CSF) analysis is indicated for evaluation of a limited number of conditions—namely, infection, inflammation, carcinomatous meningitis, multiple sclerosis, and Guillain-Barré syndrome. Lumbar puncture to measure the opening pressure is useful in diagnosing and monitoring treatment of pseudotumor cerebri and in diagnosing normal pressure hydrocephalus. For most diagnoses, the opening pressure is not helpful, but when it is needed, it needs to be obtained correctly. It is important that the patient is flat to measure opening pressure. The head should not be elevated. There should not be increased intrathoracic and abdominal pressure due to an overly compact fetal position. Once the needle is appropriately placed, the patient should slowly stretch out a bit, still maintaining a flexed posture but only a moderate one. Pressure is then measured.

Normal CSF should be clear and colorless like water. It should contain no red blood cells (RBCs) and fewer than five white blood cells (WBCs) with no polymorphonuclear cells. The report details the number of cells counted in 1 mm³ (which should be fewer than five) and then gives a percent breakdown of all the cell types seen on a spun, concentrated specimen. This percentage may include a few polymorphonuclear, and less than 30% should be normal. A WBC count of 5–10 is a gray zone that some consider normal. More than 10 cells is abnormal.

Cloudiness in the CSF is due to cells, usually WBCs, but possibly RBCs. Xanthochromia, or yellow CSF, is due to elevated protein, blood degradation products, bilirubin, rifampin, or hypercarotenemia (from ingesting large amounts of carrots).

Protein elevation in the CSF is a nonspecific marker of an abnormality, analogous to the erythrocyte sedimentation rate of the blood. When elevated, it may indicate significant disease but not point to its nature. Protein increases with infection and inflammation. It also increases with brain and spinal cord tumors or abscesses and with peripheral neuropathies. Very high protein elevations are often due to blockage of spinal canal CSF flow. Below a blockage, protein may run in the range of 1,000–2,000 mg%. At these high levels, the fluid may be gelatinous and not flow. The protein increase parallels the severity of the blockage whether due to a disk, tumor, or spinal stenosis. Protein above 150 mg causes xanthochromia. The degree of xanthochromia is proportional to the degree of protein elevation.

The tests to order on CSF are determined by the clinical situation. A cell count, glucose evaluation, and protein determination are generally considered mandatory on every spinal tap. I strongly advise against ordering Gram's stain and bacterial culture on CSF that was not obtained for evaluation of infection. Positive results are contaminants that force a repeat lumbar puncture. Venereal Disease Research

Laboratory (VDRL) tests are commonly obtained on CSF, even when syphilis is not on the differential. This is a holdover from old public health precepts. In the population at risk for acquired immunodeficiency syndrome (AIDS), however, VDRL tests, along with a cryptococcal antigen, are mandatory.

CSF analysis for carcinomatous meningitis should include a large volume (10 ml or more) for pathologic study. Generally carcinoma cells are very sparse so that large volumes must be spun down. Most of the WBCs in the CSF of patients with carcinomatous meningitis are inflammatory, not neoplastic. Since carcinomatous meningitis can be mistaken for fungal and even tuberculosis (TB) meningitis, fluid should be sent for cryptococcal antigen, fungal culture, and stain. TB culture takes 6–8 weeks to process. Its merits, therefore, depend on the situation. In AIDS patients, it is obviously of greater importance than in most other patients.

For multiple sclerosis (MS), spinal fluid should be sent for routine studies (glucose, protein cell count, and differential) plus oligoclonal bands, immunoglobulin G (IgG), and myelin basic protein. IgG requires about 2 ml, oligoclonal bands about 4 ml, and myelin basic protein just 1 ml. Oligoclonal band testing also requires blood to determine if positive bands are restricted to the central nervous system and, hence, indicates an immune response in the nervous system, or are passively transmitted from blood. In this case, a neurologist should be involved.

Evoked Potentials

Evoked potentials measure brain responses to a large number of regularly repeated stimuli to test central nervous system conduction velocity. There are four varieties: visual, sensory, auditory, and sacral. Although these are used primarily to diagnose MS, they have other, less common uses, including monitoring safety during neurosurgery. The concept is simple: A single stimulus—either a visual image, a clicking sound, or a nonpainful electric shock—produces one or more responses in the spinal cord or brain. These are too small to be identified due to random noise. Repeated stimuli are produced and the brain responses are averaged over the course of several hundred stimuli in a time-locked manner, to identify the actual response amid the noise. Averaging the responses cancels out the random noise. Most abnormalities are due to delays in conduction, but sometimes whole waveforms are missing or distorted. For MS testing, the visual evoked response (in which patients look at a television screen with an alternating checkerboard pattern) is a very sensitive indicator of optic nerve demyelination. The optic nerve remains abnormal for years, presumably permanently, after a bout of optic neuritis. It therefore confirms a second lesion in the nervous system when MS is being considered and there is no history of optic neuritis. It can determine whether a visual symptom is optic nerve–related or not. It cannot reliably interpret the severity of visual dysfunction.

The brain stem auditory evoked response (BAER) is frequently used to evaluate eighth nerve function, unrelated to MS, both for hearing and vestibular function. The somatosensory evoked response may be useful in evaluating spinal cord lesions. Sacral evoked responses may be useful in diagnosing bladder and bowel dysfunction.

All evoked responses require an intact end-organ. If vision, hearing, or sensation is severely impaired, the stimulation produces no response peripherally and thus nothing to measure centrally. In ordering the test, sensory impairment must be taken into account. All labs have parameters for determining how impaired a special sense function may be and still undergo testing.

LABORATORY TESTING OF COMMON PROBLEMS

Headaches

Few headaches are due to structural brain abnormalities. When tumors or other structural lesions cause headaches, they are invariably large enough to be seen on CT scans without contrast.

An imaging study must be obtained for an adult with new-onset or sustained headache, or for any patient with a neurologic deficit.

The only structural lesion that could be missed on a CT scan and still cause headache would be in the posterior fossa and should cause focal signs and symptoms, precipitating a neurology consultation followed by a brain MRI.

An EEG is not useful in the evaluation of headache. A lumbar puncture is only rarely indicated. If papilledema is present and the head CT scan has normal results, then opening pressure and routine CSF studies are mandatory to diagnose pseudotumor cerebri. If fever accompanies the headache and the CT scan or MRI reveals no structural explanation, such as abscess or sinusitis, then meningitis must be excluded.

Seizures

In most cases a CT with or without contrast is adequate for the evaluation of seizures, but an MRI is clearly more sensitive and occasionally reveals a tumor, cortical stroke, or arteriovenous malformation (AVM) that is missed by CT scanning. An EEG is strongly suggested. Repeat seizures do not require further investigations except in the case where seizure control had been good but was lost although anticonvulsant drug levels remained stable. This suggests an active brain process.

Stroke

Depending on what information is required about the stroke patient, an MRI may be much better than a CT scan, but for most decision making, a CT scan without contrast is adequate. When it is important to determine the number of strokes or the stroke location, MRI is clearly the better test.

Tumors and Arteriovenous Malformations

MRI is more sensitive than CT scanning for finding tumors and AVMs. However, CT scanning may be better at identifying the tumor. For example, because CT better distinguishes blood and calcium from other brain or tumor tissue, it may be better for identifying meningiomas or oligodendrogliomas because both tend to calcify.

Back Pain

The problem with routine x-rays of the back is that they are almost always abnormal except in young adults. The question becomes not whether the patient has arthritis but whether the arthritis is related to the pain. New-onset back pain requires at least one set of x-rays. Recurrent back pain does not require repeat imaging.

Radicular pain, particularly in a nerve distribution or associated with paresthesia or focal weakness, points to an MRI of the appropriate spinal segment and possibly an EMG. Spine x-rays are usually not useful. Surgeons do not operate on the spine solely on the basis of a positive EMG. The positive EMG confirms a nerve lesion and localizes it, but even in the best hands, it is an imperfect test that cannot identify an etiology. A positive MRI without an EMG may be enough to trigger surgery when symptoms are classic, but an EMG may provide evidence that the less impressive lesion on MRI is really causing most of the problem and might alter surgery.

Dizziness

Vertigo is usually a symptom of labyrinthine dysfunction and is only rarely a brain stem event. Electronystagmography (ENG) provides an objective evaluation of the inner ear. BAER is a test of the auditory and not the vestibular nerve, but because they run together, lesions of the auditory nerve may also affect the vestibular. Unless hearing is affected, the yield will be small. MRI of the brain stem is the test of choice for structural lesions, but tumors rarely cause vertigo. CT of the inner ear may be useful, but any test beyond an ENG is probably best left for the appropriate specialist, such as an ear, nose, and throat specialist or neurologist, to order.

CLINICAL PEARLS

- Evoked responses cannot be attempted on patients with severe end-organ damage (i.e., deaf patients cannot have a BAER, blind patients cannot have a visual evoked response).

- EMG is not useful for evaluating chronic neck or back pain without a radicular sign or symptom.
- CT is more sensitive than MRI for detecting subarachnoid hemorrhage.
- MRA exaggerates the severity of carotid stenosis.
- An MRI spinal survey is an excellent method of excluding spinal cord compression on an emergency basis. Sagittal cuts fine enough to detect a lesion large enough to compress the cord are made of the entire spinal cord. This reduces three separate studies (cervical, thoracic, and lumbosacral) to a single test.
- Carotid duplex should *not* be ordered to evaluate fainting or dizziness.
- EMG and EEG are only as good as the person reading the test.
- A neurologic consultation is less expensive than CT, MRI, or EMG.
- EEG is not a useful test for evaluating headaches.

Index

Note: Page numbers followed by *f* indicate figures;
page numbers followed by *t* indicate tables.